AFTER THE
WORST DAY EVER

AFTER THE WORST DAY EVER

WHAT SICK KIDS KNOW ABOUT SUSTAINING HOPE IN CHRONIC ILLNESS

Duane R. Bidwell, PhD

BEACON PRESS • BOSTON

BEACON PRESS
Boston, Massachusetts
www.beacon.org

Beacon Press books
are published under the auspices of
the Unitarian Universalist Association of Congregations.

© 2024 by Duane R. Bidwell

This book is printed on acid-free paper that meets the uncoated
paper ANSI/NISO specifications for permanence as revised in 1992.

Text design and composition by Kim Arney

*Library of Congress Cataloging-in-Publication Data
is available for this title.*

ISBN: 978-0-8070-2469-0; e-book: 978-0-8070-2470-6;
audiobook: 978-0-8070-3519-1

To Don
stellar friend and colleague

Always be ready to give an answer
when someone asks you about your hope.

—1 Peter, Chapter 3, Verse 15
of the Christian New Testament
(Contemporary English Version)

Hope is not institutional.
It is contextual and relational.
In a sense, hope is a living presence
and not a defined objective.

—Erik Freiburger,
disability advocate and voice

CONTENTS

AUTHOR'S NOTE

All of the stories and events in this book happened as described, to the best of my knowledge. Some I observed; others were told to me by children in treatment for end-stage kidney disease. I have tried to retell the stories as faithfully, accurately, responsibly, and empathically as possible, but, as I've written elsewhere, "no writer can transmit another person's stories without shaping them. A retold story never comes to readers in as pure a state as when the original storyteller entrusted it to a writer."[1] My own biases, values, and intentions shape the way I tell these stories; even when I quote children directly, you are receiving my interpretation. At times I have fictionalized a story (or parts of it) to make you engage more viscerally—seeing, feeling, hearing, smelling, tasting, and sensing what children experience. In doing so, I tried to make the stories believable, lifelike, and probable, without changing the facts or language used by children. Because children interpret things within their frames of reference, they sometimes get the facts wrong—for instance, when children say they were "in a coma," they probably aren't referring to the medical condition but to the fact that they were not conscious (which can be caused by many conditions other than a coma). My approach reflects the principles of evocative (auto)ethnography,[2] a research method that encourages scholars to tell stories in ways that evoke emotional and intellectual responses.

Children—especially sick children—are considered a vulnerable population by researchers. They require careful protection, and they don't always understand the risks involved in participating in research. All children in the book provided informed *assent* to become one of our research partners; five were old enough also to provide informed *consent*. Parents or guardians provided informed consent for the other forty-six. I have changed children's names and personal characteristics to protect their privacy, especially as they mature into adulthood. Most participants provided their own pseudonyms, which reflect idiosyncratic choices; a few asked to use their legal names, and others wanted me to assign a pseudonym to their words. Any resemblance to other people, living or dead, child or grown-up, is coincidental and unintentional.

AFTER THE
WORST DAY EVER

CHAPTER 1

TETHERED

The first time I meet William, I watch him walk through the dialysis unit like a politician working a crowd. The sixteen-year-old flashes a huge grin and greets nurses by name, shakes their hands as he passes. Each patient tethered by tubing to a dialysis machine receives a nod and a beneficent smile as William strolls the aisle between their vinyl recliners and hospital beds; kids he recognizes get a high-five or a thumbs up. Spying the unit manager at the end of the room, he spreads his arms wide and strides toward her with purpose. "Shaaaaaaaaaay-ron!" he says. "*Give* your *boy* some *loooove*!" They hug, laughing.

It's hard to believe the staff used to tease William for looking glum during treatment. ("They don't want you to look depressed or bored," he confides later. "They try to make it fun.") Today he radiates bright energy, and everyone's excited. It's been months since he visited; last year he received a kidney transplant and no longer needs dialysis.

When his doctor introduces us, William shakes my hand and looks me in the eye. "You can ask me anything you want," he says, nodding. He leans back on his elbows, propping himself on an examination table. "Anything you want to know about me, anything you want to know about anyone else, a whole lot of stuff."

A month from now, William's body will reject the transplanted kidney, sending him back to dialysis three mornings a week for nearly a year. But right now, none of us know that's coming; his blood work and examination suggest everything is fine.

William strikes me as the type of guy destined to get elected homecoming king. Neatly dressed in dark jeans and a polo shirt, he wears a gold chain around his neck, and he's articulate, poised, and carefully groomed. I can smell his cologne as he talks. William tells me he makes friends with everyone at his high school, regardless of clique; people simply *like* him, and he finds a way to connect to what they care about. His own obsessions focus on the three things he's always wanted to do: play football, join the Army, and work as a police officer. On the football field, he was one of those players coaches love because they can do it all: run, block, receive. Fast and agile, William once expected to become a local gridiron star. "I never got tackled the whole season," he says, remembering his time on the middle-school team. "Nobody could catch me. And now I can't play football again."

Three years ago, during winter break, William woke up feeling sluggish and achy. His mom thought it was the flu. All through the holidays his back and legs hurt; he slept most of the day, every day, and his legs quivered when he stood. A week after New Year's, William could barely walk. The flu doesn't cause that sort of pain, and his family doctor sent him directly to the emergency room. Tests revealed blood and protein in his urine. The ER doctor admitted William to the hospital.

"The next morning," William remembers, "a whole bunch of doctors came in. They said that I had lupus nephritis and kidney failure."

Lupus nephritis, an autoimmune disorder most common among Black Americans and Asian Americans, causes swelling, pain, and loss of function in the kidneys; it can damage them so badly that they stop working completely and permanently. When William and other people with lupus nephritis get sick, their immune systems can't tell the difference between illness and healthy flesh and blood, and their bodies attack their own cells. Protein in William's blood and urine suggested that he needed treatment right away. Three days later he started dialysis.

"That was the worst day ever," he says. "I started throwing up and stuff, and I passed out. When I woke up, I could not remember."

The hospitalization initiated a years-long routine. Three days a week, fifty-two weeks a year, William and his mom woke at 5 a.m. to drive dark streets to the hospital, where he received three hours of dialysis before going to school late. He missed a lot of class, which made it tough to keep up his grades. Sometimes, his teachers didn't believe he had health issues; they thought he was skipping school. The struggles didn't end after William received a transplant; he continues to cope with the disease and its effects, including side effects from transplant medications: nausea, dizziness, high blood pressure, diarrhea, sore joints, canker sores, rash, fever, headaches, and tremors. More than anything, William has had to reimagine his future in light of limitations. His childhood dreams seem impossible.

Millions of people have a chronic illness like William's. Nearly half the US population, including one in four children, live with at least one chronic condition: heart disease, stroke, cancer, diabetes, asthma, cerebral palsy, muscular dystrophy, and so on. About ten thousand children in the United States live with chronic kidney disease; every year, about fifteen hundred advance to the final, terminal point: end-stage renal disease. Children who begin dialysis before age fifteen usually live about twenty years after diagnosis. Those twenty years are not pleasant: End-stage disease shortens life, increases suffering, and requires patients to be tethered to a dialysis machine for hours each week. Some children don't go to the hospital for treatment but spend twelve to fourteen hours a night, every night, receiving dialysis at home. For them, sleepovers, dating, late-night social activities, and other childhood experiences are complicated—and sometimes not worth the effort.

Children develop kidney disease for a variety of reasons. Some are born with a defect that keeps their kidneys from working effectively. Others develop kidney failure due to genetics, infections, physical injury, or urinary problems such as a blockage. Others have diseases—some specific to kidneys, others that affect the entire body—that damage kidneys: high blood pressure, heart disease, allergies, diabetes, lupus, HIV, malaria, hepatitis B, hepatitis C, and more. When kidneys fail, they can no longer filter a person's blood effectively; waste products and fluids build up and cause additional health problems. Kidney disease can develop over a long period of time—months or even years. Many children with diseased kidneys have no symptoms or so few that they are not diagnosed until the disease becomes severe.

A kidney transplant remains the most effective treatment for end-stage disease. It's the only way to escape dialysis. Children with end-stage renal disease long for, anticipate, and work toward a donated kidney. Transplants are common; each month, more than one hundred US children—three or four each day—receive a kidney transplant. But a transplant isn't a cure. A donated kidney allows a patient to manage the disease without dialysis but requires daily medications and constant monitoring. After a transplant, a patient can regain some of the freedom, independence, and functioning stolen by the disease. But transplants can fail, as William learns, and when they do, a patient returns to dialysis. (William received a second transplant, a kidney from a cadaver, just before his senior year of high school after another year of dialysis.) A successful transplant functions effectively for ten to twenty years; then it needs to be replaced. Children who receive donated kidneys as infants might need two additional kidney transplants by the time they are twenty-five. Children who never receive a transplant remain tethered to a dialysis machine for hours each week, year after year, to remove poisons and fluids from their blood.

Most chronic illnesses are less severe and less dangerous than end-stage renal disease. But doctors consider kidney disease a "paradigmatic" chronic illness. That means its physical, social, and spiritual effects are shared by people with any sort of chronic condition. Knowing what it's like to live with kidney disease illuminates the broader experience of chronic illness and how sick people live well, with hope, when an illness cannot be cured. This question—how to live hopefully and well without a cure—is what I investigate in this book.

I focus on chronically ill children for several reasons. My professional roles as chaplain, pastor, and clinician often place me into relationship with suffering children. Most resources I consult about hope in suffering, however, are rooted in theory, not experience, and they privilege adult perspectives over children's knowledge. Yet children have fewer resources, less agency, and more vulnerabilities than most adults—which means the ways they cope with illness and make meaning of it are likely to be vastly different from adults in similar situations. I trust that children are experts on their experiences, and I wanted to hear what they say about hope, suffering, and illness rather than filtering what I saw through an adult lens. Doing so makes me a better care provider. In conversation with a friend who works as a pediatric nephrologist—a kidney doctor—I became convinced that sick children have something to teach us; their experiences and understandings can inform, critique, and expand adult perspectives in constructive ways. Together, we designed a study to explore how his sickest patients experience, define, and sustain hope.

Diagnosis thrusts chronically ill children and grown-ups into an unfamiliar world where they struggle to maintain physical, mental, social, and spiritual well-being. That new world demands that children and their families master medical jargon, navigate large and bewildering institutions, submit to painful and frightening procedures they don't understand, and confront the reality of death. These challenges teach sick children why hope matters and how to sustain it in the midst of chronic illness. Not all forms of hope are helpful, but the children who taught me about hope remain primarily confident, trusting, and engaged. They navigate chronic illness with relative equanimity, and their understandings of hope challenge grown-up assumptions. Their wisdom has transformed how I think about hope and how I relate with children whose lives are threatened by illness.

WISDOM IN SUFFERING?

Under William's stylish clothes, he hides a secret: multiple abdominal scars and a Hickman catheter, which doctors, nurses, and patients call a "port." The port creates a bump the size of a quarter below William's collarbone, like the knot you get on your head if you bang it against a cupboard door or get hit in the noggin by a baseball. The bump consists of a small silicone pod under his skin; a tube runs directly from the pod to William's heart. Sometimes you can see the tube bulge under the skin at the base of his neck. During dialysis and other procedures, nurses snap three smaller tubes to the port. The tubes bounce against William's pectoral muscle, and the medical team uses the tubes to draw blood and give medicine. At first, William received the catheter to make dialysis easier; nurses could attach the machine to the port instead of starting a new IV. Once he received a transplant, the port and catheter made it easier to give William medicines to support and protect the new kidney.

During his years on dialysis, William asked his doctor about a donated kidney three times a week, once at every treatment.

"So, doc," William would say. "When do you think I can get a kidney?"

"When you're ready!" the doctor would respond. Then they'd laugh.

It became a private joke, almost a ritual. But William wasn't kidding. "For me it was like this little game," he says. "I tell myself that the more you come to dialysis, the more points you get, and whoever got the most points at the end, they get a kidney."

William received the transplanted kidney two weeks before his fifteenth birthday—much faster than most people who need a transplant. Now he gets a checkup at the clinic once a month. Every day he takes medicines to manage the transplant, treat kidney disease, and address side effects. He even takes some medicines to reduce the side effects of other medications. Chronic illness cuts him off from his dreamed-of future: the fragility of the new kidney, and the catheter dangling from his chest, make rough-housing and football dangerous, even life-threatening. With his doctor's permission, William has joined the school basketball team; in a few months he'll try out for track. But serving in the military, he believes, is out of the question, and he doesn't know if he will be able to attend the police academy.

These days, though, William thinks less about the future than about his daily challenges. When other kids notice the catheter in his chest and the bulge in his neck, some point and stare; others whisper. Sometimes people laugh. William hates it. Finally, he and his cousin trapped and punched a particularly obnoxious classmate on the school elevator. After that, the teasing stopped.

"It is kind of hard to go to school and have people make fun of you," William says. "You have a catheter in your chest, and you can't do nothing about it; everybody can see it under your clothes and all that. Then when something happens at school, you'd be so scared that it would get tugged on, or it would come out." He grins. "But I'm thankful for all the stuff you don't have to do no more once you get your transplant. You don't have to wake up at five in the morning to come [to dialysis] every week!"

Most chronically ill children I've met eventually make peace with their illness, accepting its challenges as a part of life. For them, being unwell is normal. But they cannot manage their diseases alone; without fail, illness eventually stretches them beyond their capacities. They need help every day, no matter how independent and capable they feel. This can frustrate adolescents, who are developing competence and seeking independence from family. But needing help isn't the only frustration. They have myriad struggles: maintaining friendships when they can't hang out or go to parties; needing to change plans at the last minute because of symptoms or side effects or treatment delays; parsing how, when, to whom, and how much to disclose about their illness; managing the ups and downs of moods and sick bodies when there's no "typical" day; explaining scars, catheters, and bruises to curious people. Treatment itself causes suffering; it isolates children from peers and family, restricts activities, adds stress, and creates painful and uncomfortable side effects.

People with chronic illness are saturated in suffering—physical, relational, psychological, spiritual. It's easy for pain to preoccupy them and those who care for them. At the same time, people have a remarkable capacity to hope in the midst of illness. How does that happen? What sustains sick children like William when disease reconfigures their bodies, constricts their dreams, and shortens their lives? How do they stay in relationship with a body that betrays or slowly poisons them? How do they manage the limits of illness when the broader culture insists they can achieve anything if they apply themselves? And what can chronically ill children teach the rest of us about the nature and nurture of hope?

I'm convinced that clarifying the relationship between hope and chronic illness can help everyone understand how to live well with suffering—those who are ill and those who will be (because all "health" is temporary). Being unwell is a part of being human, as is coping with the limits of our bodies, minds, and spirits. Unfortunately, our political and economic systems, relational networks, and physical environments don't acknowledge that. Yet none of us can avoid suffering. Sick children, I have found, are experts at reimagining what it means to have a good life, one sustained by hope, when suffering does not (or cannot) end and when long-term futures are not assured.

Accessing the wisdom of children with chronic illness requires listening to them, attending closely to their words, and working diligently to understand what they are saying. Documenting what they know and say about hope allows grown-ups to see life-giving possibilities in the midst of chronic illness. We shouldn't exploit or justify suffering simply because we can learn from it. But learning how to identify unimagined and useful possibilities in suffering is vital, especially as climate crisis, global pandemics, and failing economic systems uncover society's fault lines and distort the lives of millions. How do we hope when despair seems rational?

RETHINKING HOPE

Like many people in the United States, I grew up confusing hope with optimism. I would say, "I hope I get that job!" or, "We hope God will cure her cancer!" when what I really meant was that I *wished* those things would happen, even without evidence that they could. I emphasized human abilities, as if hope depends on effort: "They hope to win today's race because they trained for it for so long," or, "I hope my investment in this job pays off!" This type of false hope relieves people of the responsibility to attend to reality, recognize limits, and adjust expectations in light of conditions beyond their control. Optimistic people encourage positive thinking, expect miracles, and seek guaranteed outcomes despite insufficient information, distorted facts, and a refusal to acknowledge roadblocks. They confuse hope with "progress," convinced that difficult situations can and will improve if we work hard. Especially, they think of hope as a promise: What I want will surely come to pass.

But people with chronic illness know these things aren't true. What they want in the midst of disease, what they wish for, rarely arrives. Even so they endure, love, grow, and thrive in the absence of what they desire. They live with suffering rather than escape from it. Yet as a young person I rarely thought of hope as a capacity to deal well with suffering or to live creatively with disease and its limitations. The word "hope," used casually, implies the resolution of suffering; we hope wounds will heal, and we hope traumas will disappear. But traumas endure; scars remind us of injuries. Likewise, the effects of chronic illness cannot be forgotten or erased. William will always have marks on his body from surgery and treatment, even with a healthy kidney transplant. How, then, does someone hope when suffering doesn't end and is likely to get worse? What does it mean to hope if scars don't fade or disappear? How does someone hope realistically and authentically when they face a future that includes ongoing pain and the likelihood of life ending sooner than they'd like? Children and grown-ups with chronic illness constantly face these challenges.

Authentic hope helps people thrive. It adds to the richness of life the way an orange daylily glows in a dark room, adding color and beauty: things look better, more inviting, more hospitable, even though the room remains dim. As we make sense of events, relationships, and self, hope improves health, enhances coping, strengthens relationships, lengthens life, and helps meaning flourish. Hopeful people engage more consistently at work and school. They're more productive. Hopeful children, with and without disease, find more meaning and satisfaction in life than children with less hope and children who despair.

Authentic hope can be taught and learned, and children learn it best when grown-ups do the things that strengthen a child's ability to hope—the actions that children say actually matter in the nurture of hope, as we'll explore in the rest of the book. I learned quickly that imposing grown-up theories of hopefulness on children, or emphasizing what I find hopeful as a grown-up, causes me to miss what children need. I cannot nurture hope among children without understanding what hope means to them.

Talking with chronically ill children convinces me that their hope isn't primarily about progress or a better future; it's about living well with suffering in the present. Hope doesn't correct, erase, or relieve grief, trauma, and despair; it shapes our responses to them and allows us to flourish while suffering. Despair descends when distrust, isolation, powerlessness, and disenchantment erase or limit possibilities; hope, on the other hand, feeds on trusting "something more," the possibility of possibilities. Those possibilities disclose themselves in small ways through the care and presence of the people around us, our ability to influence difficult situations, and an affirmation of life's continuity despite the losses that accompany illness. Hope manifests through the work of the Spirit, experienced as a wellspring of insight, energy, consolation, and possibility that shapes human lives, and as well as through our choice to trust the "something more" we glimpse through these experiences.

Consider Angie, a high-school cheerleader whose kidneys have failed.

DIAGNOSIS: CROSSING INTO STRANGE TERRITORY

At first glance, Angie reminds me of a baby bird fallen from its nest, trembling and terrified. She sits alone on an examination table, head bowed, staring at the floor. Her paper hospital gown falls open in the back, exposing her shoulder blades—the sort of vulnerability most fifteen-year-old girls try to avoid showing. Angie clenches her hands atop the blue blanket on her lap. Weak winter sunlight spills from a window, and the room is cold. She's been waiting a long time for the doctors and her parents to return.

Angie tells me she's scared, but mostly she wants to go home; she didn't sleep in the emergency room last night, and now she's missing cheerleading practice. "I don't care what happens," she says. "I just want to get well enough to cheer again. And I don't want to miss any more school." Then a yawn contorts her face. She blushes. "Oh my gosh," she says. "I'm sorry. I'm not usually this rude."

Lately, Angie has been tired a lot and sometimes nauseated. Her ankles swell for no reason. Ten days ago she noticed blood in her urine. She told her parents she had a urinary tract infection. She didn't tell them about the blood, and they didn't ask. The family doctor prescribed antibiotics over the phone, and Angie thought she'd get better.

Yesterday, she passed out while cheering at a basketball game. Her coach made her go to the emergency room, where doctors found protein in her urine and creatinine in her blood. Creatinine points toward deteriorating muscles. Doctors kept asking Angie if there is a history of kidney disease in her family. She doesn't know; she's never heard of kidney disease, and she's never had a serious illness. But today Angie begins dialysis, and she heard the doctor say she might need a transplant. Her mom keeps crying.

A sudden diagnosis of end-stage renal disease thrusts children like Angie and William into a world with strange customs and scary procedures. Suddenly, they're surrounded by people in scrubs and white coats speaking a dialect they can't follow. Medical jargon swirls through the air like a foreign language. People talk across their heads, almost as if the children or their parents aren't present. Nurses slip needles into veins and clip pulse oximeters onto index fingers. Vials of urine and tubes of blood seem like sacred objects, carried reverently from bedside to laboratory, scrutinized for messages as doctors seek a hint toward appropriate treatment. Children get wheeled from one frightening procedure to another: computed tomography scans, chest x-rays, blood draws, spinal taps, surgeries. No one asks what they prefer; they're just expected to hand themselves over to masked technicians wearing rubber gloves and paper gowns, wheeled away from parents toward cold examination rooms to be poked, prodded, twisted into awkward positions, and told to hold still.

The people who dwell in this land are friendly enough; they smile and laugh and tease and play, and no one intentionally causes pain or tries to scare a child. But their customs seem strange; their actions are unfamiliar, hard to trust. A child's sense of disorientation becomes heightened by an awareness of death, which envelops everything: Despite the playfulness, this culture focuses on keeping kids alive. High stakes mean serious commitment. People shift from lighthearted banter to life-saving action in a millisecond. Even the youngest children on the dialysis unit sense the reality of death and suffering; they probably cannot articulate what they sense, but it hovers at the edge of awareness. Everyone in the room knows the disease never relents. End-stage renal disease is incurable and eventually fatal, because a patient's kidneys totally and permanently fail.

The illness requires a machine to perform the functions of the kidneys, ridding the body of toxins. Healthy kidneys balance fluids in the body, regulate and filter minerals in the blood, and generate hormones needed to create red blood cells, promote healthy bones, and regulate blood pressure. Above all, they filter and eliminate waste material that accumulates in the blood from food, medications, and chemicals. Without dialysis, people with end-stage kidney disease are poisoned slowly by their bodies. No one can live long with untreated, broken kidneys.

Still, treatment only manages the disease; broken kidneys cannot be fixed or cured. Treatment can lengthen life and improve its quality, but it cannot reverse the damage done to diseased kidneys. A transplant is the best option—a new, healthy kidney to replace the one that's failed—but a transplant doesn't cure, and the side effects can be harsh. And as I've noted, a transplant isn't permanent; on average, a kidney transplant works well for no more than fifteen years. After that, the kidney needs to be replaced.

In the midst of this strange culture, disoriented by chronic illness and learning to manage lifelong symptoms, children need a way to sustain a sense of possibility, anticipation, and positive meaning. This is why hope matters. Hopeful children participate more meaningfully in treatment; they have better physical, mental, and spiritual health. Healthy, hopeful children do better in school, athletics, and relationships; they are more resilient than other children; they cope more effectively with depression and bullying, reject suicide, avoid smoking and drug use, and effectively use spirituality to cope with stress, illness, and other challenges. They are less likely to act violently. It's no wonder hope helps children with chronic illness to flourish.

UNDERSTANDING HOPE

At this point, a reasonable reader might expect me to define hope and describe how to know when children have it. I'm resisting that temptation. My goal isn't to evaluate whether children have hope, or determine how much of it, but to understand hope the way they do. That means I need to be careful about imposing grown-up concepts on children's words. Children do not experience things the way grown-ups do; their understandings are unique both to childhood and to an individual child. Too often, we take what children say and then interpret, categorize, and assess it through the lens of adulthood. We look to see if children understand things the way we do, what we consider "true," "informed," or "accurate," rather than asking what we can learn from their perspective.

In this book I try to stick closely to the statements and experiences of children. What do they mean when they use the word "hope," before they've been colonized by grown-up ideas? How do they know hope exists? What gives them evidence that hope is real? What do they say helps create hope? By apprenticing myself to children and youth, I seek to trust, honor, and respect their uses of the term—what they say it means—rather than to judge how well they meet grown-up or scholarly criteria for hoping. I want children's experiences to "talk back" to the definitions and conversations of grown-up philosophers, ethicists, and theologians. I want them to critique, expand, and revise the ways we think about hope in general.

That said, it's useful to have an idea how grown-ups—psychologists, philosophers, theologians, and others—describe and theorize hope. Knowing what the "experts" say can help us identify what children see and understand about hope that grown-ups do not.

In general, grown-ups think about hope in three ways: as an emotion, a virtue, or a set of cognitive skills. From these perspectives, hope happens "inside" a person; it's not something that can be injected or borrowed. In taking this stance, researchers assume they can understand what goes on inside someone, perhaps better than the person understands themselves. A researcher might call a particular inner quality "hope," for example, even if people themselves don't see it that way.

Grown-up perspectives on hope tend to focus on the future, suggesting that people hope because they anticipate things getting better. The future, then, is not determined in advance but open to possibilities; something can happen or become real later that isn't real or happening now. Trust in an open, flexible future allows people to set goals, identify ways to reach them, and work toward what they want. Authentic hope sets multiple goals; it recognizes limitations and takes them into account. Hopeful people aim at what's possible. They accept multiple outcomes. If their primary goal doesn't work out, they turn to and celebrate second- and third-choice goals.

But hope involves more than an ability to set goals and work toward them. It also involves an ability to imagine, see, and attend to possibilities in day-to-day life—to perceive how transcendence makes itself known in the midst of the mundane. People hope in part because they experience consolation in troubling times, moments of freedom in the midst of worries or disappointments. Freedom and consolation occur even when someone fails to progress toward their goals. People hope even in the midst of despair.

These grown-up understandings can be useful. But they emphasize cognitive, temporal, and executive abilities that children don't always have and that chronically ill people can find difficult. This emphasis limits our ability to make sense of hope in chronic illness, especially among chronically ill children. For example, children do not develop the ability to imagine and plan more than a few hours or days in advance until they finish grade school. If hopefulness depends on the ability to imagine a better and different future, then children are at a disadvantage, and young children cannot be as hopeful as grown-ups. But we know that's not true. Likewise, severe illness—especially a life-threatening illness—makes it more difficult (if not impossible) to imagine a long-term future. If hope depends on imagining a future, then people with severe illness are at a disadvantage, because disease constricts their capacity to focus beyond the present. But we also know that's not true.

In a similar way, emphasizing the cognitive dimensions of hoping—setting goals, identifying pathways, and claiming skills and resources—suggests children will be less hopeful than grown-ups because those cognitive capacities don't develop fully until late adolescence or early adulthood (if then). Chronic illness and the side effects of treatment can also impair cognitive functioning. If hope depends on advanced cognitive skills, then children under eighteen and people with chronic illness cannot hope fully. We know that's not true.

These grown-up perspectives, taken together, risk position-ing children (and grown-ups whose cognitive abilities or sense of the future are constricted) as "deficient" hopers. Because children do not perceive hope the way grown-ups do, we think their ideas about hope are immature, incorrect, insufficient, or inadequate. How often do we say to children, "You'll understand when you're older," rather than getting curious about what they already understand?

Framing hope as a virtue comes closest to matching the ways children describe hope. A virtue orients people toward what is good, motivating them to take action. A virtue is a disposition, a trait, a tendency to seek the best for self and others. In philos-ophy, hope is a human virtue; it takes effort, and people create it through repeated actions aimed at the good. Repeated actions make hope a character strength, a habitual pattern; it cannot be exhausted or squandered. In religion and spirituality, especially in their Christian forms, hope is a transcendent virtue, infused into people by God or Spirit or an ultimate realm. While people can claim and cultivate hope received from beyond themselves, they cannot create it alone. As a transcendent virtue, hope turns us toward possibilities and motivates us to work toward the good. Children, I find, experience hope as both human and transcendent, attained and received. They do not see hope as a moral good, but as an end in itself. Hope for children isn't about "right" behavior or perfection but about a receptive capacity, a trust that suffering can be transcended and that goodness asserts itself. Hope allows children to know they can be healed even when they cannot be cured.

In the end, children understand hope differently than grown-ups because their cognitive, social, physical, and spiritual capacities are still developing. But that's not a sufficient rea-son to dismiss their ideas and perspectives. We should embrace children's views as sources of insight into the nature of hope. Could it be that our more mature, more "sophisticated" capacities keep us from seeing and hearing things that children understand? When I became a student of children's lives, listening carefully to their words about illness, hope, and the ways that ordinary time discloses ultimate meaning, I learned things I don't (yet) understand.

WHY I STUDY PEDIATRIC HOPE

In many ways, my exploration of childhood hope began in the 1980s and 1990s when I worked as a journalist in Texas and India. I didn't have a particular interest in advocating for children, but my reporting frequently thrust me into that role; it was necessary, more often than I liked, to write about the harmful effects of grown-up actions on children's lives. Four stories, in particular, came to mind over and over as I wrote this book: Bubba, a hungry two-year-old beaten to death by his mother's boyfriend because the child would not stop crying; dozens of throwaway adolescents sleeping in drainage culverts and inner-city parks (and, in one case, on the roof of a suburban high school) because their parents would not allow them to live at home; unsupervised school-age children in a rock quarry outside New Delhi using dynamite and hand tools to mine rock to earn money toward a lifetime of debt incurred by their parents and grandparents—debt necessary to purchase food, housing, medicine, and the purity rites required by their religion; and articulate, bright-eyed Tibetan teenagers born in exile in the foothills of the Himalayas, yearning for a rocky plateau they had never seen but nonetheless dreamed about inhabiting in autonomous freedom.

These children were my first encounters with the nature of systemic sin and structural evil, as well as the tragic dimension of some children's lives. They unmasked precritical, North American assumptions about the "innocence" and "depravity" of children that surface when grown-ups talk about responding to these issues. Only the Tibetan children offered words and actions that hinted at the possibility of hope as a communal resource, developed and nurtured by parents, teachings, and religious communities.

I first became overtly curious about childhood hope in the late 1990s when I worked as a pediatric chaplain. My responsibilities included the emergency room, neonatal unit, and pediatric intensive care, where the sickest children receive treatment. They arrive at the hospital because of car accidents, sports injuries, sudden illness, disasters, and cancer, and I frequently talked with them from their arrival at the emergency room through hospitalization and discharge. Once I sat with parents while they told their eleven-year-old daughter she had glioblastoma, an incurable brain tumor. Sometimes I visited children in oncology isolation rooms, where they received bone-marrow transplants to treat cancer. Different children and different families navigated these crises in unique ways, and I paid particular attention to children who seemed more confident than afraid, more trusting than suspicious, more engaged than passive. I wondered what allowed them to navigate a frightening and unfamiliar situation with relative equanimity. I also saw types of hope and optimism at the hospital that aren't helpful, and I encountered the weight that shallow optimism can place on a child who feels responsible for maintaining the inappropriate and inauthentic "hope" of a family or community. Some forms of hope can harm people. That's part of why I'm writing this book.

Teaching children in congregations also led me to reflect on hoping. Sitting on the floor on Sunday mornings, telling Bible stories or hearing children's prayer requests, I marveled at the ways children can trust teachers, use their imaginations, and make profound observations about complex sacred texts. I learned that children can teach grown-ups a lot if we pay attention to them on their own terms.

During my doctoral work, I discovered psychologist C. R. Snyder's cognitive model of hoping, a powerful resource for the nurturing of hope throughout the human lifespan. The cognitive model distills hope into three types of thought: goal-setting, pathways thinking, and agency thinking. When I became a parent, I used this model to promote a hopeful attitude in our son. He and his friends became a laboratory for the cognitive skills of hoping: setting goals, identifying pathways to goals, and developing the agency needed to accomplish goals. As he learned to crawl, I put obstacles in his way—a pillow, a footstool, a stack of books—so he had to find different routes to the objects he wanted. During his preschool years, I asked him about his immediate and short-term future, encouraging the skill of goal setting. As he grew older, I tried to stretch his sense of agency and power not by doing things for him but by waiting for him to ask for help, then brainstorming strategies with him that he could implement to achieve what he was after.

Exploring hope with my son helped me identify some limits to a cognitive understanding of hope. First, it's too individualistic; it doesn't sufficiently account for the relationships and social processes that nurture hope. Second, it doesn't acknowledge how children can expand their sense of hope through the resources available in their communities; it emphasizes only the power and resources that children themselves already identify and claim. Third, it doesn't attend sufficiently to the ways children are embedded in an ecology of relationships, institutions, cultural norms, and systems of power, all of which shape hoping. Finally, the cognitive model attempts to be amoral; it doesn't provide children with resources to expand their goals beyond expectations of growth and success and an ideology that defines human worth in terms of an ability to consume. The cognitive model has political and economic implications that make me uncomfortable; it recruits children into being "efficient," "effective," and "productive" workers with a laser-like focus on goals, rather than highlighting other possible ways of being human.

As I reflected on these experiences, I started to ponder what hope looked like among children whose situations made it difficult to imagine a future, set goals, or see themselves as responsible agents. Children with chronic illness seemed to challenge ideas about hope that are assumed "true" in theology, philosophy, and psychology. Teaming with a pediatric kidney doctor, I started talking with children with end-stage renal disease—those receiving dialysis, those with kidney transplants, and those who'd been sick for a while, like William, as well as the newly diagnosed, like Angie. After spending hours with fifty-one children in dialysis units and transplant clinics across the United States, I started to understand that children with chronic illness imagine, perceive, and enact hope in ways beyond emotion, cognition, and virtue.

This insight allows me to see that children's hope has implications for what it means to be human in general, regardless of age. As I came to this realization, the global climate crisis began to dominate the world's awareness, demanding action and creating barriers to hope. I wondered whether children's insights about hope in chronic illness could help people hope in an environmentally uncertain world. Like chronic illness, the planet's environmental dis-ease amid the climate crisis truncates the future; it creates suffering, and it can be managed but not cured. We are unlikely to repair the damage done to (and by) our collective body. How, then, can we notice, sustain, and practice hoping? This broader social and historical moment shapes my understanding of pediatric hope because the experiences of chronic illness—disorientation, unpredictability, a sense of impending disaster, a shortened and limited future, and so forth—reflect in a microcosm the global experiences of people living in climate crisis. These days, all of humanity faces an uncertain and limited future—or, if not limited, at least significantly different from what we perceive as "normal." This ambiguous future intrudes on our lives and demands resiliency. Can paying attention to how children perceive and nurture hope in the midst of chronic illness help us strengthen the human response to climate crises, healthcare pandemics, and rising totalitarianism in the United States and elsewhere? Can practices of hoping help orient us in a changing world?

I think so. This book explores five practices that children with chronic illness use to sustain hope. I see these practices as resources for everyone, regardless of age or condition, who wants to remain hopeful in the midst of suffering.

PRACTICING HOPE

Children with end-stage renal disease can help us see that hope manifests through practices of community, voice, attending to Spirit, trust, and identity. These practices help them become "more normal," a phrase they use to describe what life can (and should) be despite failing bodies, shortened lives, and complicated relationships with family, friends, physicians, and disease. The chapters that follow unpack the practices, illuminating what they mean to children and for humanity as a whole. Each chapter points toward strategies for cultivating, nurturing, and amplifying hope in the messiness of life.

In the end, children perceive and receive hope in the present, and they do it through their awareness of an infinite abundance that manifests in the midst of chronic illness. This awareness allows them to say "yes" to their limitations while claiming their creativity, compassion, and trust in the goodness of life.[1] Their accounts of hope create space to re-imagine our broader understandings and to question the "thinness" of scientific, philosophical, theological, and medical understandings of childhood hope. Children's ideas point toward shifts in medicine that can make the healthcare system more about healing than cure, relationship than fee-for-service, meaning than technology. What children say confirms that hope emerges in particular places and with particular people. Efforts to cultivate and nurture hope should be custom-made for particular children and their illnesses. One size doesn't fit all.

CHAPTER 2

REALIZING CONNECTIONS

A clown in baggy purple pants waddles through the dialysis unit strumming a ukulele. She bumps hips and dances with a nurse wearing Tickle-Me-Elmo scrubs, then sees a sleeping teen at the end of the room. Looking around dramatically, the clown shifts her eyes from side to side with a sneaky grin. She holds a finger in front of her mouth to signal silence to the few people watching and tip-toes, lifting a knee high with each step, to the foot of the sleeper's bed. Suddenly, the ukulele erupts in a crescendo. The clown throws back her head and takes a deep breath. "It feels greeeeeeeeat . . . to urinate!" she crows, with a dramatic flourish. A few kids laugh. She bows, maroon hair swinging. The sleeping teen opens one eye, rolls it dramatically, then closes it again.

Most patients in the unit remain absorbed in laptops and mobile phones—listening to music, watching movies, texting friends. Others sleep. A second clown plays cards with Mark, a twelve-year-old who refuses to talk to me about hope unless I beat him at Uno. I lose seventeen games in one day, and he remains stoically silent. (I never beat him, and he wasn't interviewed for the project despite his agreement to participate and his parent's consent. Sometimes children claim power where they can!) The unit's full today, as it always is on Mondays. One empty chair sticks out like a missing tooth in a kid's smile. Christine hasn't arrived, although her appointment was scheduled to start nearly an hour ago. That happens sometimes. Both of her parents work, so she rides the Medicaid-sponsored van from home to the hospital and then to school. Sometimes the van comes early; other times, late.

This morning the van's running later than usual, and Christine's eyes are moist with unshed tears by the time she pushes through the swinging door at the front of the dialysis unit.

"I'm sorry," she says to the charge nurse. "I hate this. I would have been on time if the van came; I was ready."

Christine's last dialysis was Friday morning. Over the weekend, the toxins, minerals, and other waste products targeted by dialysis have accumulated in her blood. Sodium, calcium, acids, and potassium make her brain foggy. Her skin itches, and retained fluids make her face puffy. Her heart works harder, moving blood that's sluggish because extra fluids constrict her veins and arteries. The extra work raises her blood pressure; increased blood pressure gives her a headache. But it all feels normal to twelve-year-old Christine, who's had kidney disease since she was a toddler. Her kidneys failed in the third grade, and she spent two years on dialysis before receiving a transplant at age ten. Her body rejected the new kidney in less than a year, and now she receives dialysis three times a week.

Patients like Christine, who are late to a dialysis appointment, usually can't receive treatment; a dialysis unit runs three shifts a day, and each shift needs to start and end on time to accommodate everyone who needs treatment. But Christine's lucky: There's an empty bed during the second shift. She can start dialysis now, overlap with the second shift, and get to school by early afternoon if the Medicaid-sponsored van arrives on time.

. . . .

Children, we commonly assume, thrive on safety, security, and a sense of belonging. Predictable routines and familiar relationships create a sense of stability, which allows children to develop trust and to explore the world. Venturing beyond the well-worn paths of their family and neighborhood, they learn to identify and avoid or defuse danger; navigate unfamiliar communities and situations; and develop confidence, competence, and a sense of purpose. These skills and resources equip them for the times in life they will feel threatened, confused, and isolated. Childhood routines provide a template for responding to an unpredictable world.

But life-threatening illness jolts children and their families out of these routines, just like an unseen pothole sends a bicyclist skidding across asphalt. Diagnosis plummets children and families into chaos; nothing seems predictable, and they wander dazed and disoriented, as if in a pitch-black maze, unsure of where they are or whether they'll find an exit. Illness permeates their days, distorting time and space; horizons contract; and the intimacies of home feel distant.

Chronic illness, in particular, requires endurance. Being sick consumes time, money, energy, and dreams. Old friendships, old hobbies, and old commitments evaporate; attention retracts to *today* or even *this moment*. Coping with disease leaves no room for imagining a different future, a skill crucial to the psychology of hoping. Sometimes nothing matters to a chronically ill person but making it through the day or coping with symptoms that flare up unpredictably. Plans must be tentative and flexible; you never know when you wake up in the morning whether you'll have a good day or a bad day.

At first, people diagnosed with chronic illness see it as an interruption, a temporary pause in the action of "normal" life. They anticipate recovery, the time when the life they knew will return. But when illness doesn't go away, when a person realizes that dialysis and other treatments will last for years, illness becomes an intrusion, an unwelcome guest that ruins plans, delays dreams, and erodes abilities. With disease permanently grafted onto life, people no longer expect recovery. When this happens, it's a struggle to remember who you are apart from disease, to make sense of sickness, and establish a sense of vitality that endures despite disease. Life looks bleak: it promises an arduous trudge that goes nowhere. Children, especially, haven't developed a long view of life; it's difficult to project themselves into a future that is different from the life they are living right now.

In the territory of chronic illness, other people serve as a resting place where a child can stock up on supplies, find clean clothes, and benefit from local wisdom. A community welcomes them at the hospital, providing resources, monitoring health, offering security, and making demands. Sick children (and their families) see that they're not alone. These relationships become a primary resource for sustaining hope among sick children. When asked to describe hope, 94 percent of the children in our study named family, friends, the medical team, and other people with kidney disease; these champions create a community of support, insight, and accountability. Relationships seem especially salient to Black and Brown children; they name connections to others more frequently than White peers, and they invoke a broader range of relationships as important—extended family, elders in the community, grown-up friends, mentors, even celebrities perceived as supportive or inspiring.

Realizing connection weaves children with end-stage renal disease into a community of mutuality and trust. It makes them more confident about their medical care and about life in general. I find this significant because many, if not most, children in the world live with a "poverty of tenuous connections"—fragile, shaky bonds with extended family, neighbors, and broader communities.[1] But when sick children establish authentic, ongoing connections with people of different ages, locations, and socioeconomic classes, they are more likely to receive the guidance they need to manage illness and grow into a flourishing adulthood.[2] We learn to be hopeful from the people who surround us.

Christine doesn't wait long before a nurse calls her to the empty dialysis chair. She settles in, lowers the recliner to a horizontal position, and rolls up her left sleeve. A small purplish knot marks the spot on her forearm where doctors, years ago, surgically connected an artery and a vein with a "vascular access fistula." (Other children on dialysis receive a graft—an implanted Gore-Tex tube—that connects an artery and vein.) Arteries and veins don't usually connect; they're distinct, each with a specialized job, like the Exit and Enter doors at a grocery store. Arteries carry oxygen-rich blood from the heart to the rest of the body; the body absorbs the oxygen, and veins return the blood to the heart, where it gets pumped to the lungs for a fresh infusion of oxygen. The fistula in Christine's arm provides a durable, long-lasting spot for the placement of the two needles that are a part of dialysis; it also requires delicate care at home, and monitoring by doctors, to prevent ruptures, infections, and other complications. Even so, doctors say a fistula is the first choice when they need to create ongoing access for dialysis.[3]

For a few weeks after doctors created the fistula, Christine felt a ticklish vibration in her arm—the sensation of blood forcing itself from the larger artery into the narrower vein with each beat of her heart. Doctors call the tickle a "thrill." Over time the vein stretched to accommodate the larger flow of blood; as that happened, the thrill ebbed, and the fistula became a firm bump where doctors and nurses attach needles that connect to tubing that allow them to pump Christine's blood from her body into a machine and back again.

Today, Christine watches the nurse swab alcohol over the cocoa-colored skin above the fistula, then push in a needle. Blood immediately flows from the needle into a tube connected to the dialysis machine. Christine watches until the blood reaches the machine, then closes her eyes. During dialysis she usually feels nauseated; sometimes, she has abdominal cramps.

The nurse, finished connecting Christine to the machine, smiles. "Alright, sweetie," she says, patting Christine's shoulder. "You just relax."

As Christine "relaxes," the dialysis machine takes over for her kidneys. Inside the machine, her blood flows past a permeable membrane with dialysis solution on the other side. Waste from her blood—excess fluid, acids, minerals, and more—passes through the membrane, carried away by the dialysis solution. The blood flows back into her arm. Dialysis gradually restores the balance of fluids and minerals in her body. Each hour, every ounce of Christine's blood flows through the machine two or three times. She does this three times a week, three hours at a time. Treatment leaves her worn out and sometimes dizzy. Her vision can blur and muscles cramp. Dialysis isn't pleasant, but Christine would die without it.

Children with end-stage renal disease suffer with or without treatment, and that suffering shapes the relationships that sustain hope. Failing kidneys can't get rid of enough fluid, which causes bodies to bloat: ankles swell, faces inflate, stomachs distend. Excess fluid, coupled with excess proteins, make the eyes puffy. The heart works harder, which increases blood pressure; increased blood pressure can lead to swelling in the brain; a swollen brain creates pounding headaches. People with kidney disease sometimes feel dizzy or lightheaded, weak, and tired. Toxins in the blood build up between dialysis treatments, making concentration difficult and sleep restless. Imbalanced electrolytes cause irritability, confusion, a racing heart; as phosphorus rises and calcium falls, muscles can weaken or cramp painfully.

Patients feel better after dialysis, but "better" can be relative; treatment generates its own symptoms: nausea, vomiting, headaches, and cramps. Broken kidneys cause body parts to wear out faster, and dialysis strains the circulatory system, which carries blood to organs to provide them with oxygen and nutrients. (This strain is another reason kidney patients can develop problems with blood pressure.) By the time Christine reaches her early twenties, she'll have the heart, veins, and arteries of an eighty-year-old woman, with all the health problems that come with that. The disease does not carry a hopeful prognosis. Children with end-stage renal disease typically die as young adults.

But physical pain doesn't dominate sick children; twice as often, they talk about more insidious suffering: the existential, social, spiritual, and psychological pain of illness.

"I had a lot of catheters that were infected or went bad and stuff, and that's painful," says Rob, fourteen. "But you feel different than other kids too. Even though—you know?—you're their friend in a lot of ways. Like, you can't do things they can do, you know? You can't be like them, you know? You *can* but you *can't*. You know? It's like taking half away from being a kid—like taking part of something you do, you know, and just *taking* it, like, say, having a TV but no remote."

Rob wants to be a pediatric surgeon when he's a grown-up. The world needs more Black doctors, he says, but mostly he's motivated by a desire to connect with children.

"I know how they feel when they're sick and stuff," he says. "That's the connection, of what pain is and stuff. Some people don't understand, you know. You say it, but you might not really know. When I say it, you know I really mean it."

Illness also makes emotional and relational demands. Keeping on schedule with medicines can interrupt activities and restructure days. Peers notice limits imposed by disease. Old friends feel awkward; they treat you differently, even as new relationships—with doctors, nurses, dieticians, social workers, other patients—demand time and energy. Bodies scar. White children, in particular, say catheters, scars, swelling, weight gain, and rashes are embarrassing. When their bodies change, they see themselves differently. Peers tease them or assume they're fragile, amplifying difference and isolation. Bodies betray sick children in so many ways.

At fifteen years old, Nick was excited about returning to school after a kidney transplant. He developed kidney disease at age five. When his kidneys failed at age thirteen, doctors removed both of them to prevent infections. Two years of dialysis and multiple hospital stays left him disconnected from friends, lonely, and behind at school. A transplant, he thought, meant freedom, a return to "normal." But the surgery site wouldn't heal.

For weeks, the incision leaked pink and red fluids, and Nick had to wear "this huge diaper thing" to soak up the drainage. Even so, he decided to return to class; no one would see the diaper under his pants, he rationalized, and he could catch up with schoolwork, reconnect with friends, and rebuild his life. The first day back, during his first class, Nick felt good. He sat at a computer, absorbed in his work and enjoying the buzz of the classroom. Then his lap felt wet.

"All of a sudden," he remembers, "I just started leaking. I leaked, like, all over the chair and all over the floor. I was very embarrassed. I had to be taken out of class."

He went directly from class to the transplant clinic, where doctors closed the incision with tissue glue. For several more weeks Nick wore the "diaper thing" under his pants. Now, at seventeen, he remembers feeling more isolated after the wound healed than before the transplant. Who wants to be buddies with the kid who leaks gross stuff all over the computer lab?

YOU'VE GOT A FRIEND IN ME: MAKING CONNECTIONS REAL

Talking to children with end-stage renal disease often made me think of Buzz Lightyear, the action-figure astronaut in the *Toy Story* movies. (It's no wonder; during dialysis, many children watch one of the four *Toy Story* films on iPads or mobile phones, and I heard Buzz's tiny, tinny voice countless times declaring: "To infinity and beyond!") The films take place in a world where toys come alive when people aren't around. The toys are full of feelings, desires, conflicts, and affections. More than anything, they yearn to be played with by children, and this craving drives all their hopes, fears, and choices.

Buzz arrives, fresh from the store, as a birthday gift for a boy named Andy. When Buzz meets a roomful of his owner's playthings, he is, as a new toy, suspicious of the others; he sees himself as a solitary hero sent to save the world, and he doesn't know how to relate to others unless they are just bit players in his own story. The first film focuses on the relationship between Buzz and Andy's long-time favorite, a cowboy doll named Woody. Buzz and Woody begin as rivals, competing for Andy's attention, but they become friends and partners through various mishaps. Buzz gradually realizes his limits and comes to trust and rely on Woody and the others. He sees that toys thrive by pooling their resources; no one has everything they need, but as a team they can draw from each other's gifts and foibles to escape dangers and ensure that they're played with by children who love them. Once Buzz adapts to his new setting, the team cannot be stopped—hence the three sequels to the original film.

Just as Buzz adapted to being one toy among many in Andy's world, sick children adapt to the territory of illness. They obey the local laws, learn the unspoken rules, and identify who in the community has power. Adopting the local idiom and practicing local customs, they begin to trust the resources of the community and to share their own wisdom for the benefit of others. They get homesick for the world they knew before diagnosis, but they don't quite fit in that world anymore. Illness changes them; they must renegotiate their relationships with family and friends who don't yet understand that health is temporary, and they must rely on healthcare workers and other people with kidney disease to thrive in the territory of illness.

"It's like you have—like, you trust something," says Ryan, eleven, a transplant recipient. As a rising fifth grader, Ryan volunteers as a bat boy for a Little League team called the Cincinnati Reds. His kidneys failed when he was a year old, and he's spent a decade in the territory of illness. "Like, if you were really sick and then you went to the doctor—and you found hope in that doctor to make you better . . . because they give you, like, pills that you need or the IV—like, you have hope *in* somebody."

Ryan and other sick children know that hope is contagious—taught, nurtured, and sustained through relationships.

GETTING RESPECT, GIVING TRUST

One afternoon, months after diagnosis, Angie waited for her mom outside the dialysis unit. She asked me what other kids were saying about hope. I responded enthusiastically, sharing what I had learned. "Y'all are great teachers!" I concluded.

"We are," Angie nodded. "We could teach you guys a lot of things if you'd take the time to listen."

Too often, physicians talk *about* or *to* children rather than *with* them. When Angie started throwing up after every meal, the family doctor told her parents that she must be bulimic. "I'm not making myself throw up," Angie insisted. "I'm *sick*." She begged for a blood test, which, when finally performed, revealed her dangerously high level of creatinine, a waste product from kidney disease. High creatinine indicates loss of kidney function, which can cause vomiting and other symptoms. There are dozens of similar stories. Leigh, seventeen, suffered kidney failure due to lupus. When her doctor suggested that she was imagining pain caused by a new medication, Leigh fired him. Bradley, fifteen, pays attention to whether doctors look him in the eye and notices when they speak to him rather than to his mom.

"It makes me feel human," he says. "They listen. They don't treat me like a kid. Other hospitals—they'll treat you like you're not there; they talk to you like you're a slave or something, like you don't know anything. That's what I don't like. It makes me mad. When you're a human, you know a lot; I mean, your brain develops, you can learn stuff, you can talk. I gotta trust in what they say and what they do. They talk to me like I'm a person. That's what I like."

Sick children want to be treated like *people* rather than *patients*. They want doctors, nurses, and other grown-ups to respect them as capable human beings. They want healthcare workers to ask about their lives beyond the hospital, getting to know their families, friends, hobbies, interests, and accomplishments—and to ask about them again, at a later time. And they value caregivers who are as transparent, respectful, and vulnerable as patients are expected to be. They also want caregivers who present themselves to their patients as *people*, as well as *professionals*, by sharing feelings, asking advice, talking about their lives, and admitting when they are scared or confused. Yet caregivers, as the more powerful people in the relationship, must set the tone, must tread carefully when disclosing personal experience, and doing so requires them to listen carefully when children speak, to be curious about activities and relationships outside the hospital, to be intentional about cultivating respectful connections, and to respond to questions and predicaments with honest information.

These types of relationships, children say, communicate respect, and respect allows them to trust the people taking care of them. We know that patients who trust their doctors heal faster and survive longer than those who do not.[4] Respect builds confidence, and caregivers cultivate both by approaching children as partners in treatment rather than objects of care. This seems especially important to boys and to older adolescents.

Lee, seventeen, values how her new doctors listen.

"They actually treat me like they know what I am talking about, sometimes," she says. "That makes me feel that I actually have someone I can trust and talk to, to actually take care of me."

Children rarely reference heroic or life-saving actions when they talk about hope. They focus on small kindnesses—casual conversations, board games during dialysis, a moment with a scared and lonely child. Attitude is central; *what* team members do matters less to kids than *how* they do it. "They are not just doing their job," says twelve-year-old Max, a dialysis patient. "They are doing it out of their heart."

Children appreciate doctors and nurses who explain complicated medical concepts in everyday language; use props, dolls, and humor to explain how dialysis works; ask for the patient's impression of how treatment is going or what's beneficial about a new medication; and allow a child to choose the needle for a procedure.

"I ask questions, and they are always there to answer my questions," says Desaree, seventeen. "If they are not, I could just call just one of them up and ask them that question. . . . A lot of them will be, 'If you have any questions, here is my card, and call me for anything, and I am there.' They make me feel special, to know that I have somebody to call, . . . and I can have someone to talk to. It is nice to know that. These people, they actually give me their cards, so I could talk to them. Basically, they will try to help me out with anything. They are helping me; they are supporting me. I have hope in a lot of people."

Nick, the teen whose leaky incision betrayed him at school, concurs. At the hospital, he says, you never have to explain yourself to anyone.

"Every time you come to the hospital, they make sure that nothing is wrong," he says. "They ask you if you could need anything, and how you have been doing, and they . . . are concerned about you. They care about your family, too, and they ask, *How is your mom?* And, *How is your dad?* And, *How is your sister?* And, *Are they coming to see you today?* They make you feel wanted, they make you feel happy and loved and cared for, and they let you know that nothing is going to happen to you on their watch."

The most important way to communicate respect, children say, is to provide complete, honest, and timely information about their health and the likelihood of improvement. Children don't want positive spin or best-case scenarios; even the youngest want to know what the doctor knows, when the doctor knows it—good, bad, or indifferent. Sharing information with children implies that the team trusts them as full partners in treatment. Rather than protecting children from the truth about their bodies—trying, perhaps, to preserve an assumed "innocence"—the team gives children the information they need to make choices about their health and healthcare, implicitly acknowledging that children are able to respond and can be responsible. (Indeed, some ethicists insist that the right to understand and control one's body stands at the center of moral decision-making.) When children sense that they're receiving vague or partial information, they distrust the team, and they cannot make wise choices about their health or their healthcare. Feeling kept in the dark—not knowing or understanding medical information—gnaws at the ability to hope.

Devine, nineteen, remembers a friend in dialysis whose parents refused to share information. "She never knew what was going on with her," Devine recalls. "Her mom always knew, and her mom wouldn't tell her. She never understood why she is in the hospital. . . . You just feel better knowing. If the kids know, then they feel a little bit better."

OFFERING ENCOURAGEMENT

Roger, seventeen, waits in an examination room to see his doctor. He's wearing a soccer jersey and holding his phone, watching the highlights of a soccer game. A varsity player for his high school team, Roger received a kidney transplant four years ago. This morning's visit is routine, a monthly check-in to make sure the new kidney works the way it should. Roger feels confident; he feels healthy, his senior year starts in a few months, and he'll graduate in the spring. Next fall, he starts college. He's grateful the transplant makes that easier.

"Dialysis is something that—you are in the hospital, and you are *there*. You cannot do nothing," Roger says. "You cannot go out and eat normal food and play a sport with your friends. With my transplant, I could do that; I could be like a normal person and do a lot of stuff."

He thought a lot about hope during dialysis.

"Hope is something that you have to—you have to *know*," Roger says. "You want to have it inside of you, . . . like something to live off, to keep on going. Something that—it will give your life meaning."

What kept Roger going during the years he waited for a donated kidney?

"My family," he says immediately, breaking into a huge smile. "My family here, in Mexico, my grandparents—and all the people that told me that I could do it, make it to . . . be with them at all times. They were always with me in the good times and bad times; they were always in the hospital. They never let me down. They always support me, at all times."

Family members taught him gratitude, Roger says, and kept him focused on what was possible despite the disease. They pushed him to take his medications on time, manage his diet, and keep his body in shape—everything he needed to do to qualify for a transplant and, once he received it, to stabilize the new kidney and prevent rejection.

Doctors and nurses do a lot to hearten sick children. But children say the reassurance, guidance, and advice they receive from family, friends, and other patients are more important to sustaining hope. Parents and close family play a role in treatment at many hospitals, but children rarely perceive them as part of the treatment team. Rather, children notice the presence, encouragement, and help they receive from family members. "If you have a loving and caring family that's going to be there for you no matter what," says thirteen-year-old Gina, a dialysis patient, "then you start to feel hope."

Children repeatedly talk about their families when describing hope. They invoke parents and siblings who stay with them at the hospital and entertain them during dialysis; advocate for them with doctors; buoy them with pep talks when they are scared or sad; and help them find strength when they are ready to give up.

The best day of Andrew's life was a January afternoon during gym in his senior year of high school. He had been walking around the track by the football stadium with friends, feeling the sun on his skin, and almost forgetting about his kidney disease, when his phone buzzed with a text from his dad: "Come out to the front. We're taking you out of school."

Andrew typed back: "Why?" Then the phone rang. It was his dad. Andrew didn't even say hello. "What?"

"Come out front!" his dad urged. "They found a kidney for you!"

Andrew had waited sixteen years for a transplant. Born with kidney disease, he had been too sick to receive a transplant for most of his life. Just a year earlier, he'd freaked out during dialysis. "I don't want to come here no more!" he yelled then, trying to yank the catheter from his arm. "I'm tired of it!"

But he received a kidney one month after doctors declared him eligible.

"I thought my chance would never come," Andrew says five months later. "My family and friends kept me hoping, every day, every time, like, my chance would come to get transplanted. . . .

I just kept going, hoping my chance would come. And it came. It came fast."

People, Andrew says, make a difference in the midst of illness.

"The way to find hope is through people, through yourself, and through the people who really care for you and who are there for you from day one," he says. "They are the ones who keep pushing; they keep pushing to do things that you don't want to do, but they keep pushing . . . because they care for you, and they want what is best for you.

"I know my family loves me, and I know some of my friends love me too. . . . I don't think I would be where I am right now without my family who care for me, and my friends. . . . In my opinion, I would—I don't think I would be here, you know? Because I wanted to get—"

He pauses, then continues in a quieter voice. "So many times on dialysis, I got tired of it. So I thank God and thank my family. They kept me going."

A friend's thirteenth birthday party taught Desaree how powerful friends can be.

"There was a swimming pool, a huge one, and everyone was going swimming," she says. "I couldn't go swimming, and everybody [said], 'C'mon! C'mon!' I used to love to swim. That was my favorite thing. And now that I would not be able to swim, it kind of put me down because, like, I love swimming, but I just . . . I can't swim right now."

To swim risked an infection in her stomach catheter, which she used at home each night for peritoneal dialysis. So during the party, Desaree sat alone beside the pool, smelling the chlorine and hearing her friends laugh. She felt sad. After a few moments, her friend Alex tapped her shoulder.

"You can't swim, so I am just going to hang out with you," Alex said. She grabbed Desaree's hand, pulling her toward a nearby swing. They played together all afternoon while the other guests enjoyed the pool. "I'd rather hang out with you," Alex said, "because I understand."

Four years later, seventeen-year-old Desaree remembers the power of the phrase *I understand.*

"She had faith in me," Desaree says, "so maybe I wanted to have faith in myself. She just really cares about me; she shows that she will be there for me. . . . She just made me happy because I just—She let me know that she is there for me: instead of swimming, she would hang out with me."

Now, in high school, Alex still looks out for Desaree.

"She is always protecting me, making sure I am okay," Desaree says. "She is always making me take my medicine on time, and she is always keeping an eye on me. My parents always let me stay in her house—nowhere else but her house. Her mom is a teacher, so she knows all my medical problems too, so, my parents feel really comfortable with her. Mom still warn me about my pills—'Take your pills, take your pills!'—because sometimes I tend to forget. Now I realize, after the transplant, I can't forget, because I have to have those pills. . . . I just don't want to mess it up. So, now I am on top of my pills."

Friends remind sick children that they matter, even when they're absent.

Nick spent two months of junior high in the hospital. Doctors said he wouldn't go back to school that year. He thought about his friends all day. "In school, everybody is fine," he told himself. "And I'm just in the hospital.

"It was like I was going down," Nick remembers. "If all you think about are the negative things that are happening to you, then it seems like hope is, like, diminished. It is, like, gone."

One day the nurses put a huge cardboard box on his bed. It was addressed to him.

"My friends, my place, all my classes combined, sent me a big box of cards and mementos, Juicy Pops, and then gum and a whole bunch of stuff," Nick says. "When I got that box of stuff, that made me know that . . . I have a whole bunch of friends that miss me. Besides my family, I have a whole bunch of friends that miss me and want me to come back. They were actually thinking about me; like, they took time out of their lesson plan and out of their days to make cards and send me stuff. I mean, that means that people really do care about you. People think about you while you are gone; you have people out there that . . . want you to come back. That didn't just make my day, that made me feel so much better—I was just, like, happy the rest of the time."

Friends and family provide consistent encouragement, but sick children also benefit from multifaceted connections to a broader community. Connections with other kidney patients— children and grown-ups—are especially important. William, fifteen, worried that a kidney transplant meant he'd never work in law enforcement. Then a social worker connected him with a police officer on dialysis, and they talked about career options and how to manage kidney disease as a professional beyond the dialysis unit. Leo's new principal showed him the scar from her own kidney transplant. "I was like, 'I am not the only one!'" the fifteen-year-old remembers. "I thought it was only kids, but it is older people too. So that makes me be happy."

But the happiest connections happen over the summer during "kidney camp," a weeklong, sleep-away event for children with renal disease. (The camp, usually sponsored by a regional affiliate of the National Kidney Foundation, doesn't cost families at all, ensuring that everyone can participate.) Campers sleep in cabins, do crafts, and learn to be leaders. They ride horses, play sports, cook, go fishing, paddle canoes, hike, and climb ropes courses— everything healthy children do at summer camp. Volunteers provide round-the-clock medical care and on-site dialysis to ensure the children keep up with medications and other treatments.

Camp can be the only time children with end-stage renal disease find themselves in a majority, part of a community where everybody has scars, ports, catheters, side effects, and knows what it's like to be different. Desaree goes every summer.

"It is cool because we understand each other," she says. "We know what we are going through. . . . They just know, like, how it feels and, like, how people treat you and stuff."

MOTIVATING CARE

William, the football player who dreams of being a police officer, remembers that the first year of dialysis was especially scary. He was twelve.

"I started having anxiety attacks and panic attacks to the point where I was unhooking myself from the machine," he says. "I kept doing that, and so I went to counseling and stuff."

By the second year of dialysis, he had anxiety under control. "I got so good at not having panic attacks anymore, that I was able to talk to other people, like the new kids, about coming to dialysis. They had a new boy who came, and his name was William too. They called him Little William. He had the same problems I had, and I talked to him about how to overcome his panic attacks and stuff."

William asked the boy's parents if he could teach Little William how to use deep breathing to relax. They agreed.

"So I helped him with that," William says. "You take deep breaths without moving your shoulders or anything. You just breathe through your stomach, and that calms you down pretty fast. That helped him out."

Sick children seek connections not just to make themselves feel better but also to help others—sharing information, modeling hope, offering encouragement, and providing companionship.

Devine, nineteen, was diagnosed at age five with sarcoidosis, a rare inflammatory disease most common in her demographic—Black women. The disease causes lumps of swollen cells to grow in her kidneys, creating kidney stones. Having sarcoidosis seems to have suppressed her immune system, which led in turn to a painful rash called shingles. Year by year, sarcoidosis reduced her kidneys' functioning. She started dialysis at age nine, and she's been hospitalized at least once a year since kindergarten. During third grade she was so sick she didn't attend school at all. By now, she has a routine: The night before dialysis, she stuffs her backpack with an iPad, schoolbooks, earbuds, and a stuffed animal from her boyfriend. When she arrives at dialysis, everything she needs goes on the tray next to her bed. She likes privacy during treatment, so she pulls the curtain closed in a circle around her chair.

One morning, a child on the other side of the curtain sobbed so loud and so long that Devine couldn't do her homework. She closed her book. The child threw up, then started crying harder. "Poor baby," one nurse said to another. "First day of dialysis."

Devine remembered those first days of dialysis—how scared, lonely, and awful she felt. She pulled back the curtain to see a little girl, five or six years old, sobbing in the next bed while characters from *Dora the Explorer* giggled on the TV. The girl was all alone. "*Mamá*," she moaned, "*¿dónde estás?*"

After two years of high school Spanish, Devine knew the girl was asking for her mother.

"So I started talking to her," Devine says. "I gave her this little stuffed animal my boyfriend brought to me. It was a cat, so I said *gato*, and I started talking to her in Spanish. I made her feel better, because she had someone to talk to. The nurses gave her a popsicle, so I asked her how to say 'popsicle' in Spanish. She told me: *paleta*. She told me, '*Dora está en la television*.' So I sat with her and made her feel better."

Sick children also build futures from the connections they make during treatment, aspiring to be doctors, nurses, social workers, and nutritionists; to volunteer in the pediatric dialysis unit; and to use their lives to benefit others.

Once during surgery, Rob's heart stopped. "I could have died," says the fourteen-year-old. He wants to be a surgeon.

In the recovery room, family members gathered around his bed to ensure that he wasn't alone when he woke up. Their faces were the first thing he saw.

"I think about my family and stuff, at the moment. I saw my grandma and stuff," he says. "That gave me hope to live more, so I could be with my family. It just influenced me to do right and take all my medicine for when I get my kidney [transplant], and, you know, help other people out who are sicker and stuff, doing something good with my life. I felt like I needed to survive to help other people."

CENTERING RELATIONSHIPS, HERE AND NOW

I learned a lot over the years that I talked with chronically ill children. To understand childhood hope, I consulted those with end-stage renal disease in part because they have so many justifiable reasons to despair. It seems realistic that they would lose heart or resign themselves to sorrow, given the nature of the illness and how it influences their lives. They face good days and bad days and can't predict what will come next. They always need a backup plan, a contingency, for dealing with sudden fatigue, high blood pressure, vomiting, and other side effects. These dynamics cascade and grow more complex as years pass. End-stage renal disease, as a lifelong condition, cannot be cured. It forever changes a person's body, schedule, diet, activities, relationships, and sense of identity, and in this respect, what happens to a child with kidney disease happens to everyone with a chronic illness. I reasoned, then, that a child who sustains hope in the midst of end-stage renal disease probably has something to teach the rest of us, whether we live with chronicity or not.

That's certainly true for me. The words of the children I talked to have stayed with me; they are a source of wisdom that shapes how I sustain hope in my own life. They are part of the connections I realized over the years, relationships that model and nurture hope across space and time. At times during our actual conversations, I'd feel overwhelmed by their focus on suffering: I'd ask about hope, and they'd tell me about physical pain, scarred bodies, fears, worries, and anxiety. I'd change the subject, redirect the conversation toward hope, and they'd still describe how bad they felt. I understand now that I was one of their connections, someone with whom they could be honest about all of the dimensions of their experience—not just the positive ones but the painful ones too. Our connection was a part of what nurtured their hope.

Sometimes at the hospital I needed a break to collect myself and reflect on what I'd heard. I was always aware that chronically ill people can't take a break; I was a visitor to that world, observing but not living with the effects of illness. During the breaks, I told myself that children emphasized pain for my benefit; they wanted to make sure I understood how much they suffer before they could tell me about hope. Now I know differently. (On reflection, I'm embarrassed at how I put myself at the center of their experience, as if they were performing "suffering" for my benefit.)

Today, I understand that sick children talk about suffering because it's the place where they meet hope. They do not separate suffering and hope. They cannot. For sick children, suffering and hope are a single experience, twins hugging each other in the womb. The hopefulness of sick children emerges in the midst of pain, and pain creates the conditions in which hope reveals itself. As illness progresses and changes, children can grow healthier, more confident and more competent, taking more control over their health and coping better with illness. But they still honor suffering as the crucible for hope. How could it be otherwise?

Children confirm that authentic hope sees things clearly. It doesn't downplay pain, evil, or bad feelings; it doesn't refuse or gloss over scars or poverty or challenges; and it doesn't pretend things aren't as bad as they seem or that everything will be better if people focus just on good things. No. Hope means seeing and acknowledging hard things, paying attention to everything—all of it, good and bad—without denying anything. Learning to live with all that we feel, all that we think, all that we see, everything that happens—accepting all of it without pushing away pain or refusing to acknowledge suffering or clinging to pleasure—invites hope. Sick children talk about suffering because they see the territory clearly, and they know that hope manifests in the midst of pain. Hope doesn't erase suffering; it acknowledges it, nods and bumps fists, without putting suffering in charge. Hopefulness implies an awareness that the status quo is inadequate, that something needs to change. Hopefulness begins with clear, undistorted vision, a "courageous recognition of the way things are," while simultaneously affirming the goodness of life.[5] Authentic hope, in the words of historian Christopher Lasch, "trusts life without denying its tragic character."[6]

The longer children live with chronic illness, the more they recognize the way things are. I noticed powerful distinctions between newly diagnosed children and those who had been in treatment for a long time. The two groups think and act differently. More experienced children exude a sense of belonging, of fitting in, of knowing routines and trusting the territory of the hospital; new arrivals take weeks or months to acclimate, just like someone immigrating from one country to another. Trust and belonging emerge as children make a home in the territory of kidney disease. They come to accept—even to appreciate—living there. The initial challenge of making a new home in the midst of treatment can be a first hurdle on the quest toward sustaining hope. If children realize enough connections, establish enough relationships, to become full members of the treatment community, they live well with kidney disease. If not, their illness becomes more difficult—physically, emotionally, and spiritually. To make a home in the territory of illness—to navigate successfully—requires them to rely on the kindness of others. They need information, support, wisdom, and care from those they encounter until those others become neighbors and, eventually, friends. This requires that children be willing to embed themselves in the systems of support sustained through relationships.

Members of the treatment team are key to this process. They not only partner with kidney patients to manage the disease and its effects, in and beyond the hospital; they also create a particular culture or community that, ideally, surrounds and welcomes patients and families. The culture created by the team, especially through beliefs about health and expectations of the patient, socializes children and families into the norms of kidney disease. It provides a web of supportive resources and creates a community focused on relationships and possibilities. Children develop strong, positive, and long-term relationships, formal and informal, with members of the treatment team. When younger, they idolize doctors; when older, they treat healthcare professionals as equals, partners in a shared project, rather than as infallible experts.

The culture established by the medical team creates an ethos that influences how children develop and engage other connections in relation to kidney disease—family, friends, fellow patients, and the broader community. As a whole, these relationships—real connections—contribute to hope in three ways:

- First, children learn they are not alone in the midst of the disease. No matter how isolated from friends and communities they knew prior to diagnosis, no matter how incompetent their parents seem in the medical context, no matter how overwhelming treatment and setbacks become, children understand that they are woven into a community and medical system that offers what they need. They aren't limited by their own resources or the resources of their family; if they need something, they're usually connected to someone who can provide it. Connections assure (and ensure) that sick children need not cope alone.

- Second, connections both create social capital and contribute to inner resources that children do not have (or do not know how to access) prior to diagnosis. These resources, which are especially important for coping with the psychosocial, spiritual, and existential demands of illness, emerge through conversation, observation, mentoring, consultation, and time together. Only later do children internalize them, creating personal resources that strengthen resilience. Thus, the community holds, tends, and shares resources that help children cope with illness and sustain hope. Children need community relationships to receive and activate those resources by receiving (and often by giving) guidance, empowerment, reassurance, and encouragement. For some children, connections introduce a broader vision of future possibilities in the context of disease—for example, grown-ups on dialysis who work as police officers, other kids who successfully manage schoolwork and anxiety in the midst of illness, and professional role models who inspire accomplishments beyond the dialysis unit and transplant clinic.

- Third, by realizing connections, children and grown-ups stimulate biological and physiological responses that help sustain hope. Relationships not only help children cope, reduce stress, and feel good; they also influence children's bodies. Social interactions stimulate the body in ways that release additional oxytocin, serotonin, and other hormones that create comforting, energizing, and elevating feelings. Changes in neurochemistry also influence muscles, organs, and other parts of the body (just as bodies influence thoughts and feelings). Connections to other people promote biological healing and help restructure the brain in ways that make it easier to hope. Human connections make the body feel better, and when the body feels better, it signals increasing health to the brain; the brain's awareness of increasing health allows children more easily to think, feel, and behave in ways that support treatment, enhance wellness, and generate more hope. Strong connections to trusted grown-ups dampen despair even among children with a biological and genetic predisposition to trauma and hopelessness.

Sick children are right, then, when they say relationships create hope. They learn hopefulness from hopeful people; those relationships come before the feelings, thoughts, and behaviors that have traditionally signaled that a person has hope. Children need people who inspire, motivate, and model hope; to sustain hope, they need stable, supportive, and responsive relationships with people who care about and expect a lot from them. Sick children's insistence that hope depends on their relationships corresponds with research, which consistently shows that strong bonds with parents and other caregivers help children develop the capacity to hope. The stronger the bond, the more hopeful the child.[7] Children play an active role in the development of hopefulness by choosing to relate in meaningful ways to people they trust. But grown-ups carry the burden of establishing these relationships; it's up to them, as the people who carry more power than children, to behave in ways that realize respectful, encouraging, and motivating interactions.

This reality shifts hope from the future to the present. Relationships that nurture hope happen here and now. They are active. They require other people, and they do not depend on a child's ability to set goals, imagine a better future, or work toward a particular outcome. They depend on the ability to connect meaningfully with others in the present moment. Hope among sick children begins in the present, and it grows from the respect, encouragement, and motivation children receive from friends, family members, and grown-ups outside the family. When we see hope as primarily (or only) dependent on the future—which is the dominant understanding in psychology, philosophy, religion, education, and other areas of knowledge—we risk downplaying or ignoring the importance of connections in the present moment. Children who feel hopeful, who think hopeful thoughts, and who practice the virtue of hoping experience hope first through everyday relationships. They internalize hoping as a skill and resource they can draw on later, even when they are by themselves. Realizing connections that nurture hope, and learning to sustain them, can be a gift that children receive from their experience of disease.

In the past, I saw hope primarily as an emotional resource, located inside individuals, tied to the future, and related to thoughts that enhance agency. But children convinced me that relationships initiate and sustain hope. This allowed me to develop a more robust, complex, and satisfying vision of hoping—one tied to relationships, connection, vulnerability, and mutuality. It made me a better friend, father, husband, pastor, and teacher. It made me better at promoting more realistic and life-giving futures for people in general and children in particular. Sick children demonstrate that relationships are not the context for the work of medicine and other forms of care; relationships *are* the work of medicine and other forms of care. When relationships distinguished by mutuality, vulnerability, respect, and humanity stand at the center of care, as its goal and justification, the human ability to resist despair increases, even when despair seems warranted and reasonable.

Children, in part because of their vulnerability, remind us that we need others: Bonds of mutuality and trust in community seem central to hoping. When we suffer, we need partners rather than caregivers. The nature and quality of our interactions come first; the roles we play with each other, the functions we perform as professionals or neighbors, come second. Hope thrives in part because of the ways we accompany each other in the present. Even when the future remains uncertain or we are unlikely to achieve our goals, we cultivate and nurture hope by attending to our relationships.

SETTLING IN: ALL SHALL BE WELL

Most newly diagnosed children adapt to the territory of illness, at least partially, within a few weeks. The dialysis unit becomes comfortable, and dialysis (or other treatment) becomes a familiar ritual. They have a favorite chair for treatment and a favorite phlebotomist to draw blood; they know nurses, nutritionists, and other patients by name; and they establish a balance where illness no longer seems like a crisis, even if it doesn't seem "normal." Above all, they feel better physically. Treatment immediately tires them out but paradoxically creates more energy overall. The symptoms that prompted them to seek diagnosis ebb, and medicines improve symptoms and side effects that remain. They feel like they're getting better.

Surrounded by a healthcare team that nurtures mutual, trusting, transparent relationships, sick children begin to believe all is well: Their health has improved; they have support and resources to cope with illness; and they feel confident about managing the disease with the help of others. They imagine diagnosis and illness as temporary, an interruption or challenge that they've successfully met. Feeling equipped for what the future holds in terms of illness, now they want to move forward with school, friends, and childhood as if nothing can stop them.

. . . .

But no matter how comfortable the dialysis unit feels or how hospitable the treatment team, a child with end-stage renal disease cannot anticipate the challenges and frustrations of living with an unpredictable chronic illness on a daily basis. No amount of planning, even if a kidney transplant allows them to resume ordinary activities, can keep sick children from encountering ordeals that test their capacity to hope. How do you keep going when your body rejects a new kidney? What does hope look like when chronic illness ceases to be an interruption and becomes an intrusion? Sick children say learning to claim power in relation to the disease becomes an important way to practice hope, as we'll see in chapter 3.

CHAPTER 3

CLAIMING POWER

Hope means that you have a chance of doing something that you dream of doing, and I dream of being a normal child.

—WES, a twelve-year-old boy on dialysis

Leo and his mother sit in chairs against the wall of an examination room, murmuring in Spanish. They are waiting for the doctor. Every month they come to the dialysis clinic to make sure Leo's at-home treatment is working the way it should. The visit also allows the doctor to anticipate and prevent problems. Things can and do go wrong; twice in the past year Leo, fifteen, has been hospitalized with infections, a particular risk for his type of dialysis. But lately he feels good. He doesn't anticipate problems today.

Long and lanky, Leo plays goalie for his high school soccer team. He earns money repairing computers, mobile phones, and other electronics in the family's garage. The business is part of his master plan: First, he wants to move back to Mexico, where he was born and his extended family still lives, to play goalie in the Mexican league (preferably with Liga MX, the first division). Then he'll return to the United States for college and work as a computer engineer. Once he's saved money from engineering, he'll spend the rest of his life as a Pentecostal pastor, preaching in English and Spanish. He says he'll be able to connect with suffering people because he knows what it's like to be sick. He wants to help others the way his pastor has helped him.

As soon as the doctor steps into the room, Leo switches from Spanish to English. Speaking slowly and quietly, with a nervous smile, he greets the doctor and asks about her health. The doctor scrolls through the lab results from blood drawn a few days ago. Leo watches her intently. She frowns, almost imperceptibly, and Leo notices.

"You're angry," he says. The doctor turns to look at him.

"I'm not angry, Leo," she says. "I'm a little concerned by some of these numbers." She turns back to the computer monitor.

"What do you see?" Leo asks.

"Here," the doctor says, standing up from her chair. "Take a look and tell me what you think."

Leo slides into the chair and pulls himself close to the screen. He scrolls through lab results. The doctor smiles at his mother, who whispers, "*Que está pasando, hijo?*" *What's happening, son?* Leo doesn't answer. Finally he turns around to look at the doctor.

"My potassium's a little high," he says, "but it doesn't seem like a big deal."

"Right," the doctor says, nodding. "Your potassium's high. It concerns me because it was high last month, and it's higher now. I think I want to make a change to your dialysis. You tell me: What sort of change should I make?"

Leo thinks for a moment.

At home each night he puts three bags of dialysis solution into a machine called a cycler. Then he connects the cycler to a soft, clear plastic tube that protrudes from his belly. The machine warms the dialysis solution to body temperature, then fills his abdomen with a fluid mix of salt, minerals, and a sugar called dextrose. For a few hours, the fluid sits in his abdomen, doing the work his kidneys cannot. Potassium, phosphorus, and nitrogen from digested protein, excess water, and more flow from his body, through the membrane that lines his abdomen, and into the fluid. At a pre-set time, waste-filled fluid drains from his abdomen. Then the machine refills his belly with fresh solution, and the process starts over. This happens three times a night. Leo stays tethered to the machine twelve hours a day.

But today's lab results suggest that dialysis leaves too much potassium in Leo's blood. The doctor can correct it by adding more dextrose to the solution. Leo would probably gain weight from the extra sugar, but there's a bigger concern: increasing dextrose could damage Leo's peritoneal membrane over time—which would make dialysis less effective later.

"I think you should add a bag of solution," Leo says finally. "Four cycles instead of three, three hours instead of four. Shorter cycles will take out more potassium."

The doctor smiles. Leo's right: Instead of increasing dextrose, they could cycle the solution more often, leaving the fluid in his abdomen for shorter periods (called a "dwell time"). This would protect the abdominal membrane and make dialysis more efficient. It would also increase the stress on his body.

"Adding a cycle could be an option," the doctor says. "But I think I want to keep three cycles and use icodextrin instead of dextrose." Icodextrin, a manufactured sugar, can filter waste better during long dwell times. "What do you think?"

Leo shrugs. "It's worth a try, I guess," he says.

The doctor scribbles a prescription for the new solution mix. "We'll see what difference that makes," she says.

This interaction illustrates two aspects of childhood hope. First, by asking Leo to analyze his own lab results, name what he sees, and strategize about an appropriate medical response, the doctor invites him to claim power. Second, by engaging—accepting the invitation—Leo becomes a more active part of the treatment team. He participates in decisions about his care rather than passively receiving the doctor's wisdom. This prepares him to leave pediatric care in a few years and join the adult healthcare system. It also helps him nurture and sustain hope. Sick children say *claiming power* helps them take appropriate responsibility for managing their illness and advocating for themselves.

In general, treatment for kidney disease has four aims: preserve life, slow disease, improve quality of life, and minimize damage to other organs.[1] These goals require vigilance—exhausting vigilance. Patients, families, and doctors need to monitor how much a child drinks, what they eat, and how medications affect their bodies. Children slowly realize that vigilance and medications are now a permanent part of their lives: end-stage renal disease cannot be cured, and they will never return to a pre-diagnosis world. Living with chronic illness can be complicated, and children tend to do better when they play an active role in the process.

Claiming power allows children to set treatment goals, advocate for themselves, choose coping strategies, monitor and maintain their own health, and resist limitations imposed by disease and treatment. As they mature, they develop and exercise increasing competence in various facets of health management. They also learn to assert themselves appropriately with the interdisciplinary team, as Leo did with his doctor, as they understand better how to influence healthcare outcomes and participate meaningfully as a team member.

Children also claim power by finding creative ways to resist and cope with psychosocial pain. Some learn strategies for controlling anxiety, like William in chapter 2, who taught breathing exercises to another patient; others choose when and how to disclose their illness, and to whom. Sick children stay active in sports, music, and other activities; intentionally cultivate emotional intelligence; and shift how they relate to their bodies. Making a home in the territory of chronic illness allows them to develop and sustain the skills, resources, and agency they need to influence the illness that is now their lifetime companion.

Among the children we interviewed, 85 percent invoked claiming power as a hopeful practice. It matters most to older children, regardless of race or ethnicity, and it becomes especially salient after age fifteen. Boys in the study seem to value claiming power more than girls, especially in terms of managing symptoms, coping with suffering, and influencing the treatment team. Yet girls are more likely than boys to frame claiming power as a deliberate choice. Boys claim power unconsciously; girls say they choose to exercise it, often strategically. (These gender differences probably are not unique to chronic illness or end-stage renal disease but reflect larger assumptions about agency and power into which boys and girls are socialized by families, schools, and society.)

Over time, I've come to see that sick children benefit when grown-ups help them cultivate and claim power as a way of practicing hope. Yet children must also acknowledge the limits of power, their own and the power of others. We can never be entirely in charge of sickness. Illness has a mind and power of its own.

Sick children want to manage illness well enough to minimize their limitations and the ways disease intrudes into daily life. This is one reason they work to become a trusted member of the healthcare team, rather than a passive recipient of professional advice and services. Sick children collaborate with the team— make real connections—not just for the sake of relationship but to learn and develop the skills to manage their health. They're motivated less by a need for emotional support than by a desire to enhance their agency—their ability and capacity to produce an effect, to influence their experience—in and beyond the hospital.

Becoming part of the team gives sick children access to resources outside their families and beyond their own resilience. It allows them to draw on the expertise and experiences of various team members, to receive coaching, and to connect to networks of personal and professional capital they couldn't otherwise access. Sick children use these resources to influence and manage not only physical symptoms and effects of illness but also its psychosocial, existential, and spiritual dimensions.

"When I was littler, and before the transplant," says fourteen-year-old Etta, "my mom would be like, 'It's time to take your medicine,' and I'd be like, 'No, I don't want to take it!' because I thought it was gross or whatever. Now, after the transplant, I know I have to take it. You have to be mature. Like, if the doctor tells you that you have to start doing something, . . . you have to, like, mature and stand up and do it to make yourself better. It's more you than the doctors, really."

Understanding that managing illness is "more you than the doctors" gives some children the confidence to claim power beyond medical settings, advocating for themselves at school, at work, and even in the halls of Congress. Bradley, for example, sets firm physical boundaries with friends. With a dialysis catheter snaking from his abdomen, he knows he's at risk of life-threatening illness if the catheter gets damaged or tugged on, even playfully.

"I know my risks, and I know my boundaries," he says. "When I'm playing football, and it's too risky, I'll say no. I'll just quit and watch. They say, like, 'C'mon, c'mon!' I'll be like, 'No. I'll stay right here.' I ain't gonna keep playing and get hurt and have to go to the hospital."

Parents, teachers, and healthcare workers sometimes resist children's efforts to claim power. I suspect that's because seeing children as agents and decision-makers can conflict with two cultural stories about children: they are either innocents in need of protection or devils in need of discipline and correction.[2]

Chronic illness challenges both perspectives. Grown-ups cannot protect children from kidney disease or shelter them from its effects on bodies, identities, and the world's response to illness. Grown-ups also cannot keep children from suffering or "correct" them into behaviors that improve their health. Chronic illness requires children to be "responsible agents" who take on developmentally appropriate tasks and responsibilities.[3] Sick children can and must contribute to the common good and to their own flourishing. Being response-able nurtures hope, and sick children need grown-ups to welcome and mentor them as competent people who are capable of helping themselves and others within the limits of illness.

I watched staff members at one dialysis unit intentionally prime children to take responsibility.

Early in the morning, before the first shift, four sleepy children lined up in silence near the unit's front desk. The youngest yawned and stared glassy-eyed out the window. The other three, clad in sweatpants and T-shirts, looked sullen. One boy draped a blanket over his shoulders like a serape. Everyone avoided eye contact with the chipper receptionist, instead staring at the floor or fussing with earbuds. Across the room, two nurses and an interpreter oriented a new family. The unit, full of natural light, felt intimate, quiet, and orderly. Café tables and chairs waited on a shady balcony, where parents, staff, and patients could get fresh air and enjoy the cool morning.

At precisely 8 a.m., the first child shuffled to the desk. Sixteen-year-old Catarina picked up a thermometer, slid a sanitary cover over it, checked her temperature, and ejected the cover into a trash can. She scribbled "98.6" on the sign-in sheet next to her initials. Next, she stepped onto a scale, recorded her weight, then glanced at the whiteboard where someone had scrawled "Chair 3" by her name. Pivoting on the balls of her feet, Catarina turned toward Chair 3 and ambled over. Watching her, I thought of a bear waking from hibernation, wandering toward fresh water.

Each remaining child followed her example: taking their temperature, recording the reading, stepping on the scale, and recording their weight. It's a small thing, but these tasks make children active participants. They have a job to do at the unit; they are part of the team rather than "patients," though seeing them nestled in their assigned chairs, wrapped in blankets, feigning sleep or zoning out on their phones, they look like nothing more than children.

During her fourth birthday party, Emily complained of a stomachache. Her parents thought she'd had too much cake and ice cream. A few hours later the pain became so intense that they took Emily to the emergency room. In addition to high blood pressure and a kidney infection, it quickly became clear that Emily had chronic kidney disease. A few months later, she developed anemia, because sometimes sick kidneys don't produce enough of the hormone that tells the bone marrow to make new red blood cells. On the other hand, sick kidneys release too much of the hormone that causes hypertension, because the body attempts to increase the blood flowing through them. As Emily grew, her blood pressure kept rising, no matter what medication the doctors used to control it. Medications for kidney disease were more successful, and for seven years Emily avoided dialysis. But just after her eleventh birthday, Emily's kidney function fell below 10 percent. She was diagnosed with end-stage renal disease and started at-home dialysis.

Emily says the change to dialysis helped her see how her habits influence the disease—helping keep it in check or encouraging it to advance.

"I didn't necessarily take care of myself as much as I do right now," Emily says. "Like, I saw what it could cause, and I got scared. I didn't want that to happen to me. . . . I have to take really good care of myself, or I could get a really bad illness. . . . The highest goal I want to achieve is try to get a transplant. What I do is, I put all the bad things aside, and then I try to think of the good things, and I try and do all the good things that I think are good for me. If I don't think they are so good for me, I ask, like, one of the nurses or my mom or somebody that knows about it."

Trafford, seventeen, says claiming power means accepting responsibility for his role in treatment. "Take your meds," he says. "Do it every hour. Do what basically the doctors say. If he say you have to take it, you have to take it, and then if he says morning, day, night, breakfast hour, whatever you have to do, you would do it. . . . If you don't take the medications, you will probably get rejected [for or by a transplant]. You don't want rejection, because it is straight-up bad. So basically, just take the medications."

Rejection happens because the human immune system typically attacks anything it encounters that isn't "us"—not only viruses and bacteria but also body tissue from a donated organ. Just as the immune system resists germs, it can resist a new organ.

Trafford has a healthy respect for the possibility of rejection. He received a heart transplant when he was five months old. The medications he took to prevent rejection damaged his kidneys, contributing to lifelong hypertension. (Diseased kidneys secrete a hormone that raises blood pressure.) He received a kidney transplant sixteen years later, and now he's off blood-pressure medications for the first time in his life. He relies on exercise and diet to keep himself healthy, but he still takes medications daily to prevent organ rejection.

When children like Emily and Trafford claim power, they change their relationships to illness. They no longer see themselves as "sick kids" requiring care but as children living with a disease—a small but significant shift. "I don't look at myself as being sick," says nineteen-year-old Jewel. "I just look at it as, I have a disease. That's all. I don't sit around in the dark all day and pout or whatever; I just do everything that my sisters do. It's just something I have." Many sick children talk about disease in the third person, framing it as something outside themselves—a personified illness rather than a condition that defines them. "It's just pulling you back," says thirteen-year-old Gina. "You go forward."

Bradley, in particular, sees himself as separate from kidney disease.

"It ain't a part of me," he tells me. "I'm a part of it." He pauses to think, looking up into the corner of the room before making eye contact again.

"Well," he allows, "it *is* a part of me, but it doesn't have *control* over me. I have control of it. . . . I don't let pain or my disease take control over me. I know there's something better; I know there's something else rather than just letting it come over me. . . . I just live day by day, year by year. I don't think about the now; I think about the future—how I can do stuff . . . how I can give back. . . . I *believe* there is hope."

Bradley chooses to be hopeful despite multiple surgeries, dialysis, and chronic pain. Other children living with disease make a similar choice: They weigh the evidence, judge the trustworthiness of the treatment team, set goals for the future, and claim their ability to influence the disease. They learn to dance with its demands, rather than striving to defeat it.

Children who view their disease as an enemy tend not to fare well compared to those who view it as a part of daily life (similar to brushing their teeth or needing a step stool to reach the cereal in the kitchen). By claiming power to influence disease, rather than fighting against it, children expand their agency and freedom—aims far more realistic than trying to defeat or overcome an incurable condition. Having goals and a sense of purpose make this easier—"knowing what you want and actually being able to get down there and live life like you are supposed to," in Leo's words.

Chronically ill children name their goals and purpose in a variety of ways—"having dreams," "restarting life," "being normal." Some want to be doctors, nurses, or police officers; others yearn to teach first grade. Leo plans to work at Barnes and Noble. "That's what I want to do in my thirties," he says. "That's my long-term goal. It gives me something to think about, you know? Just a reason to be here."

Thirteen-year-old Sloan hopes to work in medicine.

"I want to be a researcher," she says. "I have to maintain good grades. I have to follow what I want to do—pretty much follow my dreams. . . . Hope to me is being able, believing, that you will be able to do what you need to do. . . . Pretty much hope is trying to make your dreams come true. Hope is like going for your dreams, reaching out to try and get them."

Some dreams and goals lead sick children to focus on the common good rather than on themselves. William, for example, turned the loss of a transplanted kidney into an opportunity to shape the ethos and policies of his high school for the benefit of other chronically ill children. He started high school after receiving a transplanted kidney. New teachers and new friends didn't know his history with kidney disease, and he felt grateful to be done with dialysis. He didn't have to be the "sick kid" at his new school, and he anticipated good things. "Hope is like 'excite' to me," he told me a few months earlier, "seeing a fun future instead of the flat present and just looking forward to the future and seeing what good things come into life. . . . Even the light is going to be different after the transplant. Yeah. It is going to be different, just more fun."

But the summer before his sophomore year, William's body rejected the new kidney. He returned to dialysis just before school started—the "sick kid" once again. Suddenly, because of dialysis, he missed a lot of class and arrived late to school three times a week. Teachers thought he was skipping.

Rather than despair, William talked to the school principal, suggesting ways to make the environment better for students on dialysis and in treatment for other diseases. With the principal's support, he gave a presentation about kidney disease at a school assembly, where he "came out" as a dialysis patient, described the disease's effects on adolescents, and outlined how peers and teachers can help dialysis patients do well in school. After the assembly, teachers started treating him differently—not as a delinquent skipping school but as a resilient and resourceful young man.

William says that researching the presentation taught him things he didn't know about dialysis, transplant, and healthcare. After the presentation, he met with his doctor to ask how best to advocate for research funding and for policies to reduce healthcare disparities. Claiming power at school led William to claim power in broader arenas.

In a similar vein, Bradley uses his experience and expertise as a patient to influence public policy. Twice, his hospital invited him to Washington, DC, to talk to members of Congress about increased funding for research and treatment.

"In a way, it's kinda like karma," Bradley says. "The hospital's given to me, and I want to try to give back. I *want* to give back. . . . I'm trying to give back, trying to get money for the hospital. . . . I want other people to know, to feel, what I feel. I believe there is hope."

When sick children talk about claiming power, they remind me of the cognitive theory that sees hope as a by-product of three cognitive skills: setting goals, exercising agency, and identifying pathways to goals. But hopeful thoughts can't accomplish everything, and children with chronic illness face significant roadblocks to claiming power. How do they remain hopeful when structural barriers like insufficient funding or lack of healthcare or inadequate insurance thwart their efforts to claim power? What resources can they access to address the ways that race, ethnicity, and socioeconomic status shape chronic illness? The world has myriad ways of limiting their power and blocking pathways to their goals.

Leo knows these struggles. He grew up with his grandmother in Mexico, where he suffered from anemia and had frequent fevers but didn't often see a doctor. Reunited with his parents in the United States at age seven, Leo slept a lot, picked at his food, and lost weight. His skin turned pale yellow, a sign of a condition called jaundice, which signaled that his kidneys could not filter enough waste from his body. Doctors said he needed a fifty-dollar blood test for diagnosis—a lot of money for a working-class family without health insurance. Eventually, Leo's mother paid for the test because the family worried about him.

Many children are keenly aware of the financial burden of illness. Fifteen-year-old Enrique, for example, a transplant recipient, defined hope as "a good job to pay for medication." Leo says kidney disease requires many sacrifices from his family; they provide the emotional and social support he needs to stay engaged with treatment, and they bear the expenses of the disease rather than buying things or saving for the future.

Leo imagines that children without these types of support feel hopeless and do not have the resources to care for themselves well enough to stay out of the hospital or qualify for a transplant. "If they don't have hope," he says, "they wouldn't do the things that help them stay hopeful and manage the disease. They wouldn't eat right and don't watch their fluids. They will go swimming; they will smoke."

Hopeful children, he says, get involved and do the things that support their health, the way he monitors lab results to track how he's doing and figure out what he needs to do—or needs to stop doing—to become eligible for a kidney transplant.

Right now, Leo's phosphorus levels are consistently high. This puts him at risk of broken bones, something he worries about during soccer. He also takes Norvasc daily to reduce high blood pressure. Leo says staying responsible for his health keeps him focused on his goals.

"It is important," he says. "You never know when you might pass away—so you would be hoping you get through this and get a kidney transplant before you pass away. And you are hoping you do all that great stuff. You are hoping . . . to get to fifty years and, like, not pass away like right now, like, when you are, like, twenty."

Most children with end-stage renal disease seem unaware of the structural dimensions of suffering, despite the ways cultural, political, and economic realities shape their experiences. End-stage renal disease disproportionately affects people with dark skin, especially African Americans—in part due to genetics but largely because of poverty, marginalization, and cultural norms that contribute to poor diets, inadequate healthcare, and fewer social and material resources to help prevent and manage disease.

Fifteen-year-old Smiley, for example, has lived with kidney disease since she was a young child in Mexico. (Her pseudonym, which she chose herself, gives a sense of her bright attitude.) When it was clear that she required dialysis, her parents decided to immigrate to the United States. Her father came to the United States first, leaving Smiley's unemployed mother alone with three young children. A year later, Smiley and her mother immigrated. Eventually her two younger brothers arrived with their grandmother.

Smiley began dialysis when she was eight years old. Her father returned to Mexico, and her mother supports the family in the United States by working long hours as a housekeeper. Smiley relies on the Medicaid van to bring her to and from dialysis three times a week. She has no control over the transportation schedule, and she's rarely on time to appointments; sometimes, she misses them. So far, Smiley hasn't been able to manage her diet, schedule, and activities well enough to qualify for at-home dialysis. But she does not focus on suffering or barriers to treatment.

"I am a normal girl," she says, grinning. "I like to go playing. . . . I would like to go to parties. I like to play with my family. I love to go with my friends, out. I go everywhere! I am a normal girl; I do whatever all normal guys do—people, normal people, and that's it. I play soccer, I play everything that I can, because I forget about me having a problem, a kidney problem, because that can put you down. And that thing does not put me down because I know I am a normal girl. It's just something tiny for me, that's something tiny for me."

"Okay," I say, challenging her gently. "But kidney disease is a big part of your life. You come here three times a week for dialysis—"

She cuts me off immediately.

"It is, but . . . it is like, well, we had to think about dialysis," she says. "When you can be something, don't think about it, and you can be happy. Forget about problems, and you can—It is like, just be yourself. And I mean, like I said, I mean, like, I feel like a happy girl because I got my family, I got my mom—she always there for me—my brothers, my family, my grandparents, and everybody. . . . My mom, when she was little, her mom showed her how to be hopeful. She . . . would be telling me the same thing her mom told her: always be hopeful, always don't put yourself down, put your head up, . . . complete everything you wish, and everything is going to come true. . . . Because, I mean, why should I put myself down when I know I am going to be okay? I got people who cares about me, I got my family,

I got my friends, I got my mom. Like I said, I got God—he is always there for me, no matter where and what I do."

Smiley envisions a clear future for herself: she will become a kidney doctor for children in Mexico. She has the intelligence, drive, and confidence to achieve this goal—as well as necessary support from her church and family—if she can receive a kidney transplant. Her brother has agreed to donate one of his kidneys to her. But because she is not a US citizen, she cannot receive a transplant until her family has enough cash to pay for the surgery.

As I leave the dialysis unit, Smiley's mother approaches me from the waiting room. Clutching a rosary, she hands me a flier in Spanish and English. It requests donations to a transplant fund.

Smiley's case illustrates the complex medical, social, spiritual, political, and economic realities that shape sick children's experiences. Many have compelling reasons to despair. Yet Smiley does not.

"Hope, for me—that is a beautiful word for me, especially for me. Hope is like me having my transplant kidney," she says. "Hope is that my mom got hope for me—my family, my friends. Hope is that someday I am going to be a doctor, like I said— kidney doctor. Someday I am going to finish with high school, college, and do everything I want. Hope is never put myself down, always put my head up and do what I can to get my strengths up. That is hope for me. . . . That means don't be sad. I will say, 'Oh my God, dialysis!' 'Oh my God, this!'—no! It is always, 'Oh, my God, I am going to do good. I am going to finish college. I am going to finish school.' Be positive, myself. Don't be negative."

There are good reasons for Smiley's dreams; Latino/a children with transplants survive longer than any other racial-ethnic group. (Black children with transplants are least likely to survive.) Yet Latino/a and Black children are least likely to receive a transplant at all; especially, they are less likely than White children to receive a preemptive transplant—a kidney to prevent the need for dialysis. This is true regardless of age, body mass, geographic location, treatment modality, or cause of kidney disease.[4] More than 110,000 people in the United States linger on the waiting list; every day, 18 of them die without becoming eligible, and every eleven minutes a new name is added to the list.

Having a living donor—family members, friends, or acquaintances who can donate a kidney—increases the chance that a child will receive a transplant. But most people in need of a transplant do not have a living donor; they need a kidney from a deceased donor, and many more people need kidneys than the number available. Doctors must carefully discern who should receive one based on health, resources for managing after transplant, stable blood pressure, effective disease management, stable mental health, absence of other illnesses, and other considerations.

Black and Latino/a children face multiple challenges to receiving a kidney transplant. They are less likely than other children to have living organ donors—family members, friends, or acquaintances—who donate a kidney to keep them alive. Their families may also have fewer resources—education, wealth, employment, and insurance—to maintain optimal health. They live with more social, economic, and health stressors that make it difficult to comply with the medical regimen required by a transplanted kidney.[5] Researchers identify a number of additional reasons for treatment disparities, including biological factors, access to insurance, immigration status, English fluency, cultural factors influencing access to healthcare, and socioeconomic status.

Poverty, especially, limits the power children can claim while living with chronic illness. The children in our study seem especially vulnerable; state and county statistics show that the rates of childhood poverty in the counties where they receive care are higher than the national average (18 percent). Two of the counties have higher child poverty rates than their statewide averages, and in those states, Black children are most likely to live in poverty. All three counties have higher-than-average rates of indigent healthcare. Average family income in the states where the children live is lower than the national average ($92,324 per year), and in two counties, the average family income is lower than the state average. Rates of high school graduation are lower than average for each county, especially among Black children, and each county has higher rates of unemployment than state and national averages.

Children with end-stage renal disease are 30 percent more likely to die during childhood than children who are otherwise healthy. Among those receiving dialysis, life expectancy stands at thirty-eight years; among those who receive a successful transplant, sixty-three years.[6] Black children have less access to transplants overall, and they are 36 percent more likely to die than other children with end-stage renal disease.[7] This is partly because most Black children are diagnosed at later stages of the disease, and partly because nephrologists are more likely to refer White than Black children for transplant.[8]

Fourteen-year-old Ebony played point guard on her middle school basketball team until a year ago, when testing confirmed that her kidneys had failed. She says hope means getting a kidney so she can play ball again. The possibility keeps her motivated to meet the criteria for transplant.

"Someone is telling you, you cannot play your favorite sport because you have an illness," Ebony says. "Makes you want to push it even more so you can hurry up and get a transplant and just play what you want to play. To be able to do that again—that is going to be a great day, it seems."

Dialysis patients like Ebony need to limit salt, calories, and foods high in phosphorus, like chicken, turkey, meat, seafood, dairy, nuts, whole grains, beans, soda, and oatmeal. Every day, they monitor how much they drink and how much protein they eat. They avoid foods high in potassium, like avocados, bananas, sweet potatoes, spinach, watermelon, beans, tomato paste, squash, and potatoes—some of Ebony's favorites. Doctors can tell when dialysis patients eat fast food, French fries, or pizza; although these treats are tasty, they elevate blood pressure and cause fluid retention. Traditional Thanksgiving meals are a curse: it seems like everything on the table contains phosphorus, potassium, and salt.

Ebony feels frustrated by all the restrictions.

"I am a very perfect kid," Ebony says, "but I do not like doing extra. . . . I can't do a lot of stuff at school. I cannot eat school food, which means I have to take my lunch every day, which means I look weird. I mean I can't do a lot of stuff."

A transplant, she tells me, will change all of that.

"I will be able to go to school every day, and I will be able to do most work around our campus. And they told me I am going to play basketball. . . . I have to work hard so I will be eligible to get . . . a kidney."

Ebony received a kidney a few months after our conversation, just before summer break. But her body rejected it before school started again, long before basketball season. Her immune system attacked the donated kidney because it was genetically different from her body. This happens to about one-third of people who receive kidney transplants. Medications can sometimes protect a donated kidney by suppressing a recipient's immune response, but doctors could not subdue Ebony's immune response. The new kidney failed.

A few months later, she's upbeat (even though she misses basketball).

"You have to stay positive," she tells me. "You never know what is going to happen. You just pray and hope that your family is there for you and just try to do whatever you can to get back on the transplant list."

Staying positive can, itself, be a way of claiming power. It helps Ebony resist the temptation of despair and identify what she can do to make sure she meets the transplant criteria again.

On the fourth day of a beach vacation, at 4 a.m., Sloan has to pee. The condo is dark, and she can hear waves. These days, she pees a lot, and it burns when she does—signs that her donated kidney isn't working well. She needs a second transplant.

When Sloan was two, her father gave her one of his kidneys. She was healthy for a decade but started feeling fatigue this summer. Her blood tests showed a steady decline in kidney function. Predictably, the transplanted kidney is wearing out after ten years. Sloan will need to start dialysis in four weeks if she doesn't get another transplant.

Sitting on the toilet, she hears her mom's phone ring. They've never gotten a call in the middle of the night, and Sloan is worried. Suddenly, her mom pounds on the bathroom door. "Sloan? Pack your bag, honey. We're going to the hospital."

A fatal car crash near home means Sloan has a donated kidney available. She and her mom drive all night to get to the hospital. That second kidney, she says, makes her excited about the future.

"Hope, to me, is being able—believing that you will be able to do what you need to do," Sloan says. "Pretty much, hope is trying to make your dreams come true—like what I still hope for. I still hope that I can take classes in college and take chemistry classes and language classes and biology classes and medical science classes, so I can do research for cures for eczema, since I have a friend who has got bad eczema, and diabetes, because I also have a friend who has got diabetes, and cancer, because my brother had a teacher who had cancer. That's what I hope for, that's what I hope to get. I also hope that I still keep doing as good as I am. Hope is like going for your dreams, reaching out to try and get them."

The new transplant doesn't make Sloan's life easy. A transplant is a lifelong commitment, requiring at least three medications, twice a day, forever, to prevent rejection. The medications increase the risk of acne, infection, diabetes, high blood pressure, weight gain, stomach pain, diarrhea, hair loss, swollen gums, bruising, and cancer. But Sloan says those possibilities are better than rejection.

Catarina knows about organ rejection. She received a new kidney two years ago, but her health got worse instead of better. Alport syndrome, a genetic disorder, complicated the transplant. Doctors worked hard to prevent rejection, including replacing her own plasma with donated plasma every week. But the new kidney didn't survive, and Catarina returned to dialysis.

"It is okay," she tells me. "Just a life learning, all over again. I will still be better, and I can do better. I still want to reach my dreams, so I cannot just let that bring me down and stop the whole world. I don't like it, but I don't let that stop me. When I found out I had kidney disease, first question I asked: Was I going to die? But mom told me that I can live with it and still have a life with it, so that's what I did. . . . I believe that I will get a [second] transplant and take care of it, and I can still go out and do the stuff that I wanted to do and still have a life to me. I am not going anywhere."

Sick children often talk about doing what they want to do, having a life, like other kids. They call it "being normal." Sometimes they talk as if they are somehow "less than" peers—deficient, distorted, or broken because of chronic illness. For them, returning to "normal"—or close to "normal"—becomes a primary goal. But who decides who or what sets the bar for "normal"? Whose interests are served when a child perceives herself as "abnormal"? How are ideas about "normal" imposed and policed at home, at school, at the hospital, and in the broader culture? What are the consequences of not being "normal"?

In the beginning, I heard talk about "being normal" as oppressive and harmful. I bristled internally every time a sick child compared themselves to what counts as "normal"; in my mind, it set an impossible standard, one that chronically ill children could never measure up to or achieve. But as I listened, I began to understand that sick children invoke "normal" as a sort of preferred vision or possibility. They don't see themselves as "abnormal"; they see "normal" as an ultimate hope.

Etta, for example, maintained hope through years of dialysis. Five years after getting a kidney transplant, she's doing well; she says the possibility of transplant gave her hope. I'm curious about her experience.

"What was it about knowing you could get a transplant that made you more hopeful?" I ask.

"Just knowing that I could be kind of—that I was—normal, that I would be more normal," she says. "When . . . they set the date for [the transplant], I was, like, really happy and stuff, just 'cause I knew it was here. It was time to get it, and I could get it over with."

"Move forward."

"Yeah."

We're quiet for a moment, sitting in an examination room at the transplant clinic where Etta gets a checkup twice a year to make sure her body isn't rejecting the kidney.

I broke the silence. "You said, 'I was normal, but I'd be more normal'?" Etta nods. The question lingers.

"What is 'more normal'?" I ask.

"Like, not always have to worry," Etta says. "Like, 'Keep your shunts in or you will end up in the hospital.'" She rolls her eyes.

"Before the transplant," I say, "you always kind of lived with that: 'Anything I could do could end me up in the hospital'?"

"Yeah." She nods.

Every child on dialysis hopes for one thing: a transplant. They want it, they dream about it, and they work for it. A transplant offers freedom from dialysis, from diet restrictions, and from curtailed activities. It allows them to participate in life like other kids, without being tethered to a machine. Given these promises, sick children quickly learn the medical criteria for receiving a new kidney, and they work diligently toward those standards— monitoring labs (like Leo), managing their diet (like Ebony), and making sure they take medications on time (like Trafford). Team members coach them into habits that increase the likelihood of qualifying.

It seemed logical to me that children on dialysis want a new kidney. But the more I listened, the more I realized that a transplant isn't their ultimate goal but a pragmatic step toward a larger vision. In their words: being normal.

Paolo, sixteen, received a preemptive transplant two years ago. For six years he managed kidney disease with medication, but his kidney function started a rapid decline when he was twelve, and doctors wanted to avoid dialysis. The best part of the transplant, Paolo says, was avoiding the restrictions, stress, and social effects of dialysis.

"Now I do everything like a normal person," he says. "I am a normal person; that's what the kidney transplant did. I could do almost anything, just take care of my kidney, . . . drink my medicines, drink lots of water, exercise, eat well, and, yeah: I can do everything. I have to take care of myself, that's all."

When sick kids invoke "normal," they're not saying they want to be like everyone else. They don't necessarily see themselves as more deficient, distorted, or broken than others. "Normal," for them, refers to a state of well-being, the ability to live in ways that realize their potential, reduce stress, do fruitful work, and contribute to the community without being cured—what the World Health Organization calls "health."[9] "Normal" can be a child's shorthand for a vision of the future that they'd prefer to live in.

The idea of being normal (or "more normal," to use Etta's phrase) provides children with a vision of what can be, rather than what is. It motivates them to claim power. It orients their energy, imagination, and creativity toward a more abundant life. They know they might never fully reach it (especially given the long-term challenges of life with a kidney transplant), but it still inspires them. It's a vision of what's possible, a preferred future less constrained by the limitations of disease. As an ideal vision, normal critiques life-as-it-is. The lure of "normal" keeps sick children engaged in improving their situation. Sometimes, hope motivates people to maintain the life they have, rather than work to improve or allow the illness to cause a decline. But for sick children, hope in "normal" entails making life better.

They also describe a more immediate experience that communicates what they value about being normal. This is an awareness of a nonmaterial abundance that surrounds them day by day. They experience it the most when they're with family, friends, and supportive members of the interdisciplinary team. This abundance is tied not to a particular outcome or goal (even a "good" outcome) but to an awareness of something more—what contemplative teacher Cynthia Bourgeault calls an "immediate experience of being met, held in communion, by something intimately at hand."[10] Bourgeault names this "The Mercy," an awareness or presence that generates strength, joy, and satisfaction. The abundance present in normal moments seems to motivate sick children to claim power. It gives them confidence in the goodness and value of life.

Smiley, for example, describes dinner as the most hopeful moment of her day. She beams, talking about being gathered around the kitchen table with her mother, grandmother, and brothers to pray before the meal. The experience serves as a touchstone for her; it grounds her throughout the day, providing a reminder of God's presence with her and with her family (a dimension of hoping that we'll hear more about in chapter 4). "Nobody knows God," Smiley says. "So I don't know what he looked like. The only thing I know: always have him in my heart since the day I was born. That's what I know—that God always be there for me."

Other sick children describe similar moments—hanging out with friends, playing video games with a mentor, planning for careers and relationships that acknowledge but are not determined or limited by disease. These moments motivate them to continue claiming power in relation to the disease and to the wider world.

"Hope is keeping up," says Tom, eighteen, a transplant recipient, "looking forward, being happy and joyful while you still can, looking to the bright side of life and enjoying life and your family—all the good things in life. . . . Just hanging out with my friends and family and looking to the bright side of life—all the good things in life. Thinking I am eventually going to keep this kidney transplant."

It's a trust in the goodness of life, a willingness to keep going without giving up.

In 2017, I was diagnosed with lymphoma, a blood cancer. After several months of treatment, the doctor declared me cancer-free, and as I recovered I decided that jogging could help me regain strength. Earlier in life I swam, hiked, biked, and competed in tae kwon do (a Korean martial art), but I hadn't exercised regularly since my thirties, so I was cautious. I started my running program slowly to build endurance and condition my weakened, obese body. Predictably, I injured myself. After a physical therapist examined my swollen foot and ankle, she put her hands on her hips and shook her head. "We need to find you another sport," she said. "Most people aren't built to be runners in the first place. Even if they are, they don't start in their fifties."

I'd hit a limit related to my age, my sedentary habits, and my biology. (When I was twenty, one doctor tried to dissuade me from activities that stress the knee by saying, "You have Subaru knees on a Cadillac body." I still have Subaru knees, but now my body is more like a Dodge Caravan: built for comfort, not for speed.)

All humans, even those who are temporarily healthy, encounter and cope with limits. We are constrained by our biology, family, social contexts, cultures, and more; not everything is possible, no matter how much we want it. I thought about this a lot when sick children told me they yearned to be normal. Is that an attainable goal? No matter how much power sick children claim, there are things they cannot change or influence; they will always be "abnormal" to some degree. Even when a transplant frees them from dialysis, it imposes certain limits. A rejected transplant rudely reminds a child of the impossibility of the "normal" they imagined. What happens when they realize that "normal" is an ever-receding horizon? How do they stay hopeful when "normal" proves unattainable? Can they learn that the limitations of disease aren't a blemish or an enemy but an expected (and normal) part of being human?

These questions become salient to anyone who lives with disease as a lifelong companion. The perpetual challenges of chronic illness cannot be resolved. Accepting this truth requires perspective, empathy, and dialogue, as well as a shift in how a person understands and relates to illness. Children who learn to accept their illness look for pragmatic solutions to ongoing challenges rather than seeking once-and-forever victory over disease. They pick their battles, stop trying to change the illness, and invest energy in things beyond their own health struggles. They seek to understand the illness rather than push it away or hold it in contempt. They feel more empathy for themselves and others, and they seem less driven by the idea of normal than by a desire to make a difference in the world. When they shift from "hope for myself" to "hope for us," it's almost as if they see chronic illness not as an adversary but as an ally—a source of wisdom, insight, and compassion. People with chronic illness not only *suffer*; they also *gain* wisdom, compassion, insight, and more. Identifying and claiming these gifts can be another way sick children claim power. Often they respond by turning outward, trusting life, and investing energy and power into practices that participate in abundance and generate goodness. Like disabilities scholar and activist Sami Schalk, they might say: "Disability is not a catastrophe to me. It's just a fact of life."[11]

Listening to and seeing the ways that sick children claim power convinces me that goals and visions are central to nurturing hope; this element of contemporary understandings of hope resonates with children's experiences. At the same time, as noted in the previous chapter, hope cannot be located solely in anticipating the achievement of future goals; it requires action and relationships in the present. The role of here-and-now relationships in helping children claim power points toward one way that children challenge recent understandings of hope. They treat hope as more than an individual effort based on a person's sense of agency and ability to set goals. Rather, hoping becomes a group project; learning to claim power requires shared social capital. Children learn from grown-ups and peers how to access, claim, and strengthen their influence. They know that people need to help each other claim power.

Hope also grows exponentially when children develop an active awareness of a "something more" that manifests spontaneously, here and now, in rare moments. Hope cannot be separated from context, as if it were a universal human experience. Prescribing Smiley's vision of abundance, for example—dinnertime prayer with family—is unlikely to generate hope for William; likewise, William's vision of a school where teachers and peers understand and accommodate the challenges of kidney disease cannot be prescribed to Leo. Hope dances to an indigenous beat. It emerges from the soil, weather, cosmology, and culture of particular times and places; it is both progressive and chronological and tied to specific locations and situations. Hope occurs in the places, relationships, and events that reveal abundance, who and what we can be at our best; it is tasted, seen, felt, and smelled, digested, danced, tilled, and shared.

The longer children live with chronic illness, the more they recognize their role in generating, sustaining, and responding to hope. More experienced children claim power more often; they convey confidence, and they act in ways that anticipate and mimic the "normal" they seek, even if they can't quite reach it. They see clearly what is, and they anticipate a fuller and more fruitful future.

Sick children are right when they say claiming power nurtures hope. They learn hopefulness when they see themselves able to influence the present and the future. Experiences of influence help them dream of what might be possible, and they consequently think, feel, and act in ways that signal they have hope. Children need grown-ups who nurture them as responsible agents; they need jobs to do, tasks to carry out, and accountability for meeting expectations. Claiming power can be a gift that children receive from their experience of disease; it increases a sense of freedom and unveils possibilities in the midst of limitation. By identifying and plucking those moments when they can influence the disease and the world, children awaken to an abundance present in any given moment.

I suspect that the practice of claiming power also gives sick children resources to avoid feeling despair when they encounter limitations they did not expect—when they realize they can never completely, or constantly, be "normal." When that vision proves insufficient, they claim power by turning to relationships and working to influence their situation, confirming that they are "good enough" even when imperfect and when "normal" feels far away. This experience shifts children inward; no longer focused on making connections or claiming power in the material world, many discover that attending to Spirit—affirming, empowering, consoling—can become an important practice of hope, as we see in the next chapter. (I am using "Spirit" to point toward the transcendent dimensions of life—what some call God or "The Universe" or non-dual reality.)

CHAPTER 4

ATTENDING TO SPIRIT

Without God, I really can't do it. It is a lot of burden on somebody my age.

—EBONY, a fourteen-year-old dialysis patient

I talk to God like he is my friend, and so I just pray.

—GRADY, a fifteen-year-old transplant recipient

Twice in the same month, thirteen-year-old Roger got matched for a kidney transplant. Both times, he hurried to the hospital, and both times doctors halted the surgery. The first kidney wasn't an optimal match; the second had an abnormality that made it impossible to transplant. Yet Roger says he wasn't disappointed because he didn't expect a transplant to happen either time. "At that time, I didn't think that I will get a kidney," he says. "I felt that it was not a good time—or at that time it was not *the* time—to get my kidney."

Months later, asleep on the living room sofa, Roger was jolted awake by a 3 a.m. phone call. He answered before his parents. "Roger?" said the hospital's transplant coordinator. "We have a kidney for you. Can you come to the hospital?"

This time, Roger had no doubt that the surgery would happen. He woke his parents and headed to the car.

"I felt like hope," he says, "like I will get my kidney, and that would be—it was going to be—a good kidney for me. And it was."

He credits a dream for his confidence.

"I always told God that one day I will get my kidney," Roger says. "Before I got my transplant—before—I always dreamed with God. I was dreaming with him, and I remember that he told me that—he showed me a kidney, like, in my dreams. He showed me a kidney. He showed me a kidney, and he told me that was *my* kidney. And like, a week later, they called me—like, 3 a.m. in the morning—and I went, and I got my transplant."

Suffering of any type, and especially the suffering of children, sparks hard questions: How could a loving, caring, merciful, present, powerful God allow young people to suffer this much? If God exists, why do children this young face such a threat to their lives? Who or what causes suffering, and how do we overcome it? At heart, these are existential and spiritual questions. Children ask them in particularly personal ways: Why is God doing this to me? Did God give me kidney disease because I'm bad or did something wrong? Am I being punished? Why won't God heal me?

When I first started learning about hope, I was surprised that few researchers mentioned religion and spirituality. People rely on spirituality during difficult times, and positive religious coping—collaborating with God, forgiving others, perceiving God as benevolent, feeling God's presence in the midst of suffering—leads to healthier and more effective responses to trauma, abuse, and other negative experiences.[1] (Negative religious coping—blaming God, seeing illness as a struggle against demonic powers, despair about one's ability to influence God, feeling abandoned by God, and more—leads to less salutary outcomes.) But secular researchers seem to ignore the relationship between hope and Spirit; everywhere I look, they attribute hope to any-thing but spirituality and religion. I'm not certain why; it could be discomfort with the language of spirituality and religion or a failure to recognize it when they hear it. It could be the difficulty of dealing with the issue of suffering from spiritual and existen-tial perspectives. They give attention to philosophical virtues, social support, cognitive skills, positive emotions, and coping strategies, but beyond the academic discipline of theology, few explore how people's spiritual and religious commitments shape hope. Even Christian theologians who talk about hope focus more on philosophy, doctrine, and psychology than personal spiritual experiences and practices.

Yet children reference religion and spirituality again and again when talking about hope, and spirituality influences the other hopeful practices that children employ. More than two-thirds of the young people in our study say attending to the presence and action of Spirit helps them sustain hope. They talk about prayer, about a certain feeling that reassures them, about sacred texts and prayer beads and chaplains and religious leaders. They say they receive reassurance, comfort, and consolation from a transcendent source that helps them remain hopeful, whether they call that source God, Spirit, The Ancestors, The Universe, or something else. This presence makes itself known during dialysis and on dark, lonely nights in the hospital, reminding children that they are not alone but accompanied by an ultimate reality, a benevolent energy that witnesses and relieves their suffering, participates in their treatment, and strengthens them in the midst of illness. Some children talk about an anthropomorphic being or higher power; others describe a compassionate, numinous reality that can be felt rather than seen, cradling all of life and working for good, whether humans notice it or not.

Connecting to Spirit seems to be a skill and resource that sick children bring to chronic illness. It's not something that emerges from the illness but is something cultivated long before diagnosis through their relationships with families, friends, and faith communities. Children rarely volunteer this aspect of experience to healthcare workers and other professionals. But if you ask about it, or simply follow up when they mention "God," they engage eagerly.

Twelve-year-old Max, for example, a transplant recipient, told me how God used his ancestors to give him confidence.

"When I found out I had kidney disease," Max says, "God said, 'Son, this is going to pass; nothing is going to stay; it is going to pass.' I prayed, and he tapped me on my shoulders and told me not to worry about anything—be a normal kid."

Later, he learned that doctors would remove his kidneys. "When they told me I was getting my kidneys taken out, I said, 'How can I live without kidneys?!'" he remembers. That night, his deceased great-grandmother, a West African immigrant, came to him in a dream. "My great-grandma—in the spirit—she is in my dreams, talking to me. That is when I found out it would be okay." He says God spoke through this ancestor.

"I thank him [God] for telling me that," Max says, "because I thought I was going to die. He told me, 'You are not going to die,' [that] he is going to be the one to take care of me, and I am going to live—and don't worry."

For children like Max, actively attending to Spirit marks a shift in the ways they cope with and sustain hope during illness. Immediately after diagnosis, they turn outward, realizing connections with the treatment team and claiming power in the healthcare system and in relation to the disease. But eventually they learn that connections and power alone do not sustain hope. No matter how many connections they make, there are times they still feel alone; no matter how much power they claim, they cannot change or influence everything. In particular, the vision of "normal" that motivates them to imagine new possibilities and work toward health cannot be realized through their own efforts. "Normal" exceeds their capacity to create, and they begin to sense they will always be "abnormal" to some degree. Even a transplant imposes limitations, and a rejected transplant slaps a child awake to the impossibility of the "normal" they imagined. Aware of loss, fearing death, and recognizing human limits, many sick children respond by turning toward an inner, transcendent source of affirmation, empowerment, and consolation. By attending to Spirit, sick children sustain hope when human power isn't enough and "normal" remains beyond reach.

Turning to Spirit might be a universal instinct among sick children. For most, it's a kinesthetic experience; they sense Spirit with their entire being—body, soul, and mind.

"All kids have that one feeling that, you know, when you're there [feeling it], it's just, you want to smile or something," says thirteen-year-old Gina, a dialysis patient. "You just want to be there, and you just get that nice, relaxed feeling—feeling relaxed all the time. . . . God is always there for you, even when you don't think he is here."

Around the world, a vast majority of people aged twelve to twenty-five say life has a spiritual dimension, and they describe it in similar ways: believing in God, believing in purpose, being true to your inner self, and being a moral person.[2] In a worldwide study of eight thousand youth, almost 40 percent of participants described themselves as "very" or "pretty" spiritual.[3] They see spirituality as relational, intrinsic, intentional, and woven into daily life—just as children in our study view hope. They say family members are the biggest influence on their spirituality, with nature, music, solitude, and service to others also playing a role. Given the results of this major study, then, I wasn't surprised that sick children say attending to Spirit generates and sustains hope.

Among children I spoke with, girls and boys attended to Spirit in equal measure, but the practice seems especially important among Black and Brown children. Eighty-five percent name attending to Spirit as an aspect of hope, compared to 15 percent of White children. This is consistent with data that indicates Blacks and Latinos in the United States are more likely than Whites to pray, believe in God, and say religion is important to their lives.[4] Other studies indicate that spiritual well-being plays a greater role in navigating illness among Blacks and Latinos than among Whites.[5]

Across all racial-ethnic groups in our study, the theme of attending to Spirit—which I identified by analyzing our conversations with children—received nearly as many mentions as the theme of realizing connections, and twice as many as the themes of claiming power, choosing trust, and maintaining identity. Children who attend to Spirit talk about it a lot, making it one of the most robust practices identified by our research.

Of course, "attending to Spirit" can mean a lot of different things, as can the terms "Spirit" and "spirituality." I am writing about the ways that children express their faith in the world—the attitudes and actions that define their relationship to a transcendent goodness, however they understand it.[6] Spirituality shapes a person's image of God or ultimate reality; it informs the way they pray, how they connect and attend to Spirit, what they believe about serving others, and the importance they place on community.[7] A person's values—what they are and how they are enacted—emerge from their spirituality. In short, I am using the concept of spirituality here the way Joan Chittister, a Christian Benedictine nun, describes it, as "the filter through which we view our worlds and the limits within which we operate."[8]

Some scholars talk about spirituality as consisting of the way we make meaning, our sense of communion with something greater, and having a purpose in the world.[9] I certainly see these elements among the children who talk with me. Children *make meaning* by clarifying values, creating a coherent vision of reality, and deciding what they believe about the basic, fundamental nature of reality.[10] They engage questions of identity, values, and existential choices to order, structure, and find significance in their experiences.[11] *Communion* in spirituality refers to a person's sense of connection to something larger than themselves, and children describe feeling the presence of God or Spirit—including a sense of being invited or called to benefit others. *Purpose* relates to the overarching direction of a person's life and the contributions they want to make to the world. Sick children express altruistic impulses, seeking to channel what they've learned from illness into care for others in similar situations.

As I tried to understand what children meant when talking about God, prayer, sacred texts, the presence of The Ancestors, and more, I often recalled a description of spirituality offered by my friend Joseph D. Driskill, a scholar of Christian spirituality. He says spirituality has three characteristics: it's shaped by a person's communities and relationships, sustained by their practices, and embodied in their moral and ethical actions. The ways people talk about and express spirituality can reveal a lot about their assumptions about ultimate reality, what it means to be human, and the relationship between the two.

Listening to people describe their spiritual understanding, including children, provides a glimpse into their attitudes toward reality. Some people describe Spirit as distant or even separate from the world; others think it acts directly in the world and in their lives. Some people talk about Spirit from an experiential or kinesthetic perspective, as Gina does; others talk about Spirit from intellectual or ethical perspectives. Assumptions about Spirit lead some people to engage with the world and with relationships, while others are led to separate themselves from people and from worldly involvement. As I listened to children in our study talk about Spirit, I tried to identify their assumptions: Does this child believe humans can hear and see God? If so, how? How does another child think people should listen for guidance from transcendent sources? What spiritual disciplines or practices—prayer, pilgrimage, art, music, rosaries, sacred texts—are useful to particular children, and how do they engage them? What does this child assume about how God thinks, acts, and feels? What about the characteristics of ultimate reality?

I found that children with chronic illness describe consistent ideas about Spirit, its characteristics, and its interactions with them and with the world. In particular, they talk about hope's connection to faith, God's character, and prayer. We'll explore each in turn.

FAITH

Riley started coughing a few days after her fourteenth birthday, and her parents thought she had a cold. But it didn't go away. Eventually, after a steroid treatment, the cough stopped, but Riley started throwing up—once or twice a day at first but sometimes as many as five times. Two months later, on the Friday after Thanksgiving, her parents took her to the emergency room. Her kidneys had failed.

Riley's body makes antibodies that attack her lungs and kidneys. It's an effect of Goodpasture syndrome, an autoimmune disorder. While the lungs of people with the syndrome don't usually sustain long-term damage, their kidneys can quickly swell and eventually fail. This damage cannot be reversed. The syndrome, rare among children, can be fatal without quick diagnosis and treatment. Riley nearly died before doctors identified her illness.

At diagnosis she was admitted to the intensive care unit, where she had a seizure. She stayed there for a month, undergoing chemotherapy to suppress her immune system and slow the attack on her kidneys. "I was just, like, very scared," Riley remembers. "I told my mom, like, 'I feel like dying, feel like I'm going to die.'"

But then she felt a presence in the intensive care unit. She and her mom saw a tall, beautiful angel in the corner of the room. The angel was praying and infusing Riley with healing energy.

"You could feel his presence," Riley remembers. "It was not such a fabulous-great-exciting feeling, but it was calming. It was peaceful. And it was absolutely no fear."

Now, six months later, she goes to the hospital four hours a day, three times a week, for dialysis. She says no matter what happens, God will keep her going because she has a purpose.

"I have hope through God," she says. "God didn't take me this far just to let me die. . . . I know that God put me in this position so I can make a difference in people's life, just a difference in their world. I know this is for, like, reasons. So I keep hope, knowing that every day I am going to survive. . . . Just kind of knowing that, like, through my whole life—that is why I have so much faith in God. . . . No matter what, it is like I am going to make it through because it is there; he has got me."

Faith, she says, gives her confidence.

"When I was first in the hospital, like, me and my mom would always say, like, 'I am not scared,' like, 'I am not fearful. . . . I am not scared of this,'" Riley says. "Whenever I was, like, going in for surgery, I was not scared. It was just like, this was just normal, like God is just like holding me, and . . . I could feel that everything was going to be fine. . . . It was just like an emotion—just like my whole body was just, like, wrapped around, like, him, just feeling, like, comfort."

Like Riley, other children who attend to Spirit, girls especially, say hope depends on faith—faith in God, in Goodness, in others, and in possibility. Many talk about expecting miracles as an element of faithfulness. Yet theirs isn't a "blind faith," trust in something they've never seen or experienced. Rather, they validate and sustain their faith through concrete evidence that things can and do get better, even as the effects of chronic illness continue to cause suffering. As proof of Goodness, sick children point to positive laboratory reports, rising energy levels, activities they can do again (or for the first time) after treatment, and support from friends and families. They don't need miracles, physical healing, or magical transformations to prove Spirit's presence and action; they attend to tiny advances, small positive changes in health, attitudes, feelings, and relationships as evidence of Goodness, and their faith increases. Sometimes, it's as simple as seeing that members of the healthcare team expect improvement and trust that it will happen. If doctors believe, so can children.

For the children I talked to, faith isn't a capacity they develop, something that comes naturally from within. Rather, it is a gift from the Ultimate itself, however they understand it; whatever its name, it is a goodness at the heart of reality. Spiritual practices— prayer, service, ritual, reading sacred texts—primarily *express* faith and secondarily *encourage* it. Practices are a response to the gift of faith, not a way to claim it, and they're a way of staying in relationship with Goodness.

This type of faith carries children through trials. They trust things will get better, and they fall back on this belief when they face tough challenges. They remain positive and happy, they say, because they have faith that things can and will improve. There's a steady element of *trust* in the words kids use to talk about faith. Faith doesn't eliminate their trials or negative feelings; children emphasize that you can be scared, angry, and hopeless, and still have faith—and they say that not everyone is aware of faith, even when they have it.

"You are hopeful," says thirteen-year-old Sloan, the girl who received a second transplant during a beach vacation. "You get this kidney because you know that God created you for a purpose, so you want to fulfill that purpose. You have hope that you can—by hoping you can get a transplant. That's pretty much all contributors [to hoping]."

Some children in our study talk about faith as a feeling, an internal state; what they say expresses a trust in possibilities both finite (like a transplant) and transfinite (like a supreme being or eternity in heaven). Trusting in transfinite realities seems to help them maintain hope for finite goals. In fact, some children suggest that transfinite faith precedes hope; for them, spiritual awareness is a condition for experiencing hopefulness.

"God is here with us," says Leo, fifteen, after the appointment where his doctor asked him to interpret his laboratory results. "If I die, I am okay with God. . . . But, like, some of the kids, they have hope but they don't have faith. They are scared to die. . . . No matter what, having hope and faith—they will be until you die and lose everything. . . . My faith is that I have faith in God, and he will help me with, like, transplant; he will help my mom to get the money for kidney transplant."

Children also say God helps them find donors for transplant. Riley, for example, says her faith in God led her to type "kidney donors" into Google during her first week of dialysis. One email later, she had signed up with a faith-based website matching potential donors with patients, and within weeks three people had agreed to be tested for compatibility. Riley expects to receive a transplant after less than a year of dialysis. She sees God's hand in that.

"I always felt like I am going to be, like, waiting on the list," she says. "I knew that God would, like, bring me someone. . . . I was just—I mean, if you want to donate a kidney, why not go on Google, find somebody?"

There's a definite social dimension to faith. When things are tough, when faith ebbs (and many children believe faith can be "lost," although most talk about loss of faith being a matter of degree rather than presence or absence), they turn to prayer and to family to help maintain their faith in God and the possibility of an improved future. They especially turn to this support when they feel less faithful than in the past. Riley, for example, prays with others via Facebook and receives supportive text messages.

"My mom and the kidney donors text me every day with Bible verses," she says. "It's, like, crazy because I have . . . been on dialysis for only seven months, and some of these kids have been here for so much longer. It is like I can't believe this process is going by, like, so fast."

Social support helps sustain faith among sick children. But the object of their faith is a transcendent reality, a benevolent partner most call God.

GOD

Tall and slender, fifteen-year-old Enrique sprawls in a chair at the transplant clinic, thumbs dancing on PlayStation controls while digital FIFA players kick a soccer ball across the screen. For a decade, doctors managed his kidney disease with medication; for most of childhood he didn't think about being sick. He played with his cousins, roughhoused on the basketball court, volunteered at church, and hung out with friends. But a year ago his kidneys suddenly failed. Doctors told his parents to put him on the waiting list for a transplant. He'd need dialysis until a kidney became available.

"My mom signed me on Friday onto the [transplant] list, and then they called me on Saturday, the next day—just one day—and they gave me the transplant," Enrique said. "It is like a second chance. Hope is like something, like, you have a feeling that you are going to accomplish something, they are going to give you something—they are going to give me a kidney, and I would not go on dialysis."

He wasn't surprised by the speed of the transplant, because, he says, all of his life something bigger than himself, his family, and his church has watched out for him.

"Sometimes you have a feeling, like, you are protected," he says. "You are wondering that nothing [bad] is happening to you—like you have God or an angel or something; you get the feeling that something is protecting you and all that. . . . When you have that feeling . . . I think it was like God or something, an angel. Sometimes I feel it . . . , and sometimes I just know."

Children like Enrique don't just have "faith"; they express faith *in* something. They tend to call that something "God," but they experience it through events in the world, synchronicities, and a confidence that a power works for good on their behalf. It's a personal power—one that stays in relationship with them, communicates, and sometimes sends messengers like angels, ancestors, and physical sensations that provide comfort, consolation, and confidence. Above all, that power—God—hears and responds to their concerns.

"Everyone should be able to talk to God," says Nick, now seventeen. "They can talk to him right here. You may not have seen, or you may think, 'He is not hearing me.' But he hears all of us. He heals you too—physical—and he heals you in emotion. He heals you anytime, in a way that you think you need."

Children who attend to Spirit talk about God in consistent ways: God is good. God hears their prayer. God listens to them. God can be felt and known through their bodies. God lives in them and acts on their behalf in the world. God watches over them. And God makes demands, asking them to participate in healing rather than waiting for God to do it all.

"He is like the voice in your head," Nick adds. "He is the voice in your head that says, 'I am going to make *this* happen, but in order for me to make that happen, *you* have to make *this* happen.' So he told me, 'In order for you to get this kidney, you have to be patient and live your life as if you have two kidneys.' And I did. I said, 'Okay, I am going to do that.'"

This relationship, though, isn't all puppies and rainbows. Children trust God, and they blame and rage at God. They describe a dynamic, give-and-take relationship with Goodness; God, for some, becomes an intimate friend—the *most* intimate and trustworthy friend ever. They can be honest with God, and so they are—they say they *must* be honest with God—because God remains faithful to them no matter how they feel or what they say.

This becomes important to children as they ask the types of difficult questions that haunt some suffering people: Why did I get sick? Why is this happening to *me*? Am I sick because I'm a bad person? Is the universe punishing me or teaching me a lesson? If God is good, why does suffering even exist? If God can do anything, why haven't I been healed? Do I deserve this pain? If I pray hard enough, will I get better? If I don't get better—or don't get a transplant or don't tolerate my new medication or don't get through dialysis without feeling like crap—does that mean I've disappointed God? Am I getting sicker because I'm angry? Why isn't treatment working?

No one who believes in God can fully resolve these spiritual and existential dilemmas, of course—at least not adequately or forever. But feeling safe and accepted enough to express these types of questions to God goes a long way toward helping sick children (and grown-ups) cope with physical, spiritual, and psychosocial suffering.

"When I had the kidney disease, before I was on dialysis, and even when I was, I used to—honestly—I used to blame God," says eighteen-year-old Andrew, a transplant recipient who's had kidney disease since infancy. "I kept asking God, 'Why can't I be like my friend, to be healthy and not go through this and just not all, be on these meds and catheterizing all the time?' . . . I would tell myself that I was tired; God was punishing me, but I would never know why or what he was punishing me for. I would never know why. . . . I thought he was punishing me because I had kidney disease, my grandma died, then my sister died in the same year. I thought he was punishing me, taking the things I loved away. He was punishing me for something, and I just never knew what."

Andrew shared his bitterness with his parents and with a church member. The church member prayed with him and suggested a Bible verse about Jesus casting away evil. As Andrew reflected on the verse, things started to change. Being honest about the anger, he says, allowed God to respond and speak to him through sacred text; the verse helped him imagine how life would be when God repaired what evil had put him through. "It gave me more hope," Andrew says. "God was giving me a brighter light to walk in. Since then I got the transplant."

Nick shared a similar reflection directly with God. He thought constantly about needing a kidney transplant, and the longer it took, the more frustrated he became.

"Honestly, I was like, 'Did you hear me at all? I prayed, but what happened?' But he did; he just took a while, that's for sure. . . . I think he was upset with me because I was upset with him, and he said, 'Until you let this go, I am . . . not going to let you suffer, but you are just going to have to wait even longer.' . . . He says patience is a virtue, and when I was upset with him, I thought about saying, 'No, it is not a good idea.' I mean, he is God after all; you shouldn't get upset with him. And then I said, 'No, I am sorry; this is not a good idea. I didn't mean to get upset. I am sorry.' And that was it. I let it go. I didn't have a reason to be upset. . . . He created us in his image, so in a way he is one of us—in a way. So, I feel like I can talk to him like I will talk to anybody else . . . as a friend, as a really close friend."

Thirteen-year-old Audrey, a Mormon, also gave God a piece of her mind when her kidneys failed despite dialysis. She and her family read scripture and prayed daily, asking for a blessing, a donated kidney.

But when the kidney came, doctors canceled the surgery because of a problem with the donor's blood.

"I was totally frustrated," Audrey said. "I just got so angry. I got frustrated. It seems to me that nothing worked, that God was not helping me."

Audrey and her family prayed every day, asking God for a blessing. One day, her dad asked why she was so mad.

"I told him that my kidneys were not functioning. [God] is not helping me," she says. Her dad explained the transplant process and urged her to continue praying—especially for the person who would donate a kidney for her someday.

Audrey received a transplant a few weeks later—evidence, she says, that God does bless her and will bless her in the future.

"I thought it was not going to come true, but it did come true," Audrey says. "At first I thought [God] didn't exist, but from that, he does exist. . . . It did help me a lot, and he has blessed me a lot, and he has been taking care of me and being safe and healthy for my kidneys."

What does she carry away from that experience?

"Believe and trust God," Audrey says. "Believe and trust God. Don't be afraid. Don't be afraid. I pray and trust, and that helps."

Audrey's reliance on prayer reflects a third element of attending to Spirit: children with chronic illness use prayer to connect to Goodness and to express and sustain their faith.

PRAYER AND RITUAL PRACTICE

Prayer, especially prayer with other people, is the primary way sick children attend to Spirit. They pray in community with members of their church, mosque, synagogue, or temple; they pray at home and over the phone with aunts, uncles, grandparents, and siblings; they pray digitally with strangers, friends, and other kidney patients via text, Facebook, and other venues; they pray with religious leaders, privately and in public; and they pray alone in their hospital beds at night. They pray about their illness, and they pray for others. Engaging in prayer comforts sick children; it calms them, clarifies their feelings, and keeps them connected intentionally to Spirit. Prayer becomes a way of claiming power and influence in relation to the divine and to issues that transcend illness.

"Praying gives me hope to believe that God will bless you through [the illness]," says nine-year-old Maggie, a transplant recipient. "Believe that God will bless you through it, no matter what happens. I pray before I eat and go to bed, every day. I pray before I go to my classroom. He blesses me with the [health] issue I had, and he is going to bless other people with the issues they have." She especially prays with the donor of her transplanted kidney, an aunt who teaches her to attend to Spirit in the midst of everyday life.

But sustaining that attention isn't easy. Prayer slips away in the midst of busyness, and awareness of God can evaporate in the pain and stress of treatment.

"I have definitely felt more, like, of [God's] presence than I have ever had before," says Riley, a dialysis patient introduced earlier in this chapter. "It is kind of, like, hard. It is hard to stay [aware of God] because I am just, like, constantly—like things are going on, and it is really hard to, like, stay focused on God and, like, pray and go to church and stuff. . . . But when I do have, like, times to just, like, pray and stuff, it is just like I am sorry that I am never, like, there, like, talking to him. But when I do have the time, it is just like . . . It is great because I really do like feeling him, you know? Like, I have never felt him like that before. . . . It is a knowing feeling, right? It is just like you know it in your head; you know that everything is going to be fine, and you feel like everything is going to be fine in the end. . . . God didn't take me this far to just let me die; like, . . . if I am going to die, it is going to be like—I don't know—like, when I die it is going to be, like, when I am old. Because I know that after this I am going to—I really want to—do something. Like, I want to do something like counseling, or I want to be part of, like, [the] Make-a-Wish Foundation. I want to make a difference in people's lives and stuff."

For sick children, prayer isn't only speaking to God, asking for help or for guidance. It also involves other ways of connecting with Spirit: clutching a rosary or fingering prayer beads during dialysis, volunteering to help others in and beyond the hospital, wearing religious jewelry, worshiping with others in community, reading sacred texts, singing gospel music, visiting prophets and fortune-tellers and *curanderas*, and taking part in rituals. When fourteen-year-old Amber, for example, goes to the transplant clinic, she wears her grandfather's mother-of-pearl cross. When he died, she asked her grandmother for the necklace, and feeling the cross against her skin reminds her of her grandfather's strength during his own cancer treatment. "He used to wear it when we were out with him and when I went to the doctor," Amber says. "It reminds me to have faith. To me, [hope is] something like faith."

Sick children know many ways of praying and expressing faith. "Some people pray loud, some people pray in their head, some people pray during dinner," says seventeen-year-old James, a transplant recipient. "But me—don't matter 'til now—I scream, I cry when I am praying. I need the help."

What James and other children with kidney disease describe about attending to Spirit fits with psychological understandings of religious coping, the ways that people rely on religion and spirituality to navigate crises, challenges, and strong emotions.

RELIGION AND COPING

Spiritual and religious coping consists of actions, feelings, thoughts, and relationships that help people make sense of life, and deal with it, in the context of the sacred. "Sacred" here refers not only to God, divinity, or higher powers but to any dimension of life that a person recognizes as carrying transcendent or divine meaning. The sacred provides a sense of connection, transcendence, and meaning in life.[12] It provides a filter or lens for making sense of experience. Because of these functions, religion can be a powerful psycho-spiritual resource during stressful events, including chronic illnesses and treatments like dialysis—as we saw with Riley's sense of God's presence, Audrey's emphasis on prayer and trust, and Wes's healing collaboration with God.

Spirituality not only shapes a person's relationship to the sacred but also their ability to experience intimacy with others and their sense of identity, control, and transformation.

People who use religion positively feel securely related to a transcendent force; they feel spiritually connected to others, and they see the world as a safe, benevolent place.[13] They look for a strong connection to God, actively seek God's love and care, collaborate with God to put plans into action, identify how God strengthens them in particular situations, ask for forgiveness, and turn to spirituality to stop worrying about problems.[14] People who engage in these activities have fewer psychosomatic symptoms in the present and show spiritual growth in the future. Negative coping for these people involves behaviors like wondering if God has abandoned them, feeling punished by God, questioning God's love, wondering whether their religious community has abandoned them, attributing events to the devil, and questioning the power of God. People who use religion in this way show increased psychological distress and symptoms, a poorer quality of life, and greater callousness toward other people.[15] From a psychological perspective, these negative ideas could "reflect underlying spiritual tensions and struggles within oneself, with others, and with the divine."[16]

Children who say that attending to Spirit nurtures hope demonstrate both positive and negative religious coping. Some, like Andrew, feel that God uses illness to punish them for some unknown offense; others, like Wes, feel abandoned by Spirit, believe God expects impossible things from them, or worry that insufficient faith leads to rejection by God. Yet religious coping is rarely all positive or all negative; usually it's both at once, and at any given moment falls on a continuum between the two poles—more negative or positive but not entirely one or the other. Andrew, for example, thought God was punishing him (negative coping) but turned to his religious community, prayer, sacred texts, and meditation to overcome that limiting and harmful belief (positive coping). Among the children who talk with me, though, religious coping tends toward the positive, making it a vital resource for hope in the midst of chronic illness.

At its best—toward the positive pole—religious coping reduces anxiety,[17] empowers people on dialysis,[18] and increases an ill person's ability to care for themself. Bringing spirituality into dialysis, according to medical research, can reduce stress, improve quality of life, enhance sleep, reduce fatigue, and increase compliance with treatment; it can also improve spiritual wellness, enhance self-esteem, and strengthen feelings of agency.[19] Numerous studies correlate spiritual well-being with a person's capacity to hope.

When psychologist James Garbarino and his colleagues studied children in war zones around the world, they learned that children's spirituality protects them from the effects of trauma—and that children who interact with grown-ups whose spirituality gives meaning to suffering ultimately cope better with violence than those who lack such relationships.[20] If spirituality can be a protective factor in the midst of chronic violence and chronic trauma, why wouldn't it be a hope-sustaining resource in the midst of chronic illness?

Diamond, seventeen, had felt isolated most of her life. She grew up in a military family, and the Navy moved her dad around a lot. That meant changing schools every year or so, which made it hard to make friends. Plus, Diamond's primary illness, the autoimmune disease lupus nephritis, often kept her out of school—especially after it affected her kidneys.

She'd known since elementary school that lupus could cause kidney problems, and three parts of her life increased the chance of that happening to Diamond: she was young, Black, and female. Her kidneys failed by the time she turned twelve, and doctors removed them surgically. Diamond started dialysis, but a surgery led to an infection; the infection led to a seizure, which left her nonresponsive for weeks. She spent three months in the hospital. The whole time she was unconscious, her aunts and grandmother made sure at least one person prayed beside her bed around the clock.

Diamond says faith and prayer sustain her hope—that and knowing God will never abandon her.

"You have to have faith that God does stuff for reasons," she says. "He takes you through things so you can be a testimony to somebody else. You get through whatever . . . you are going through. You can tell people how—like people that are going through something similar or the same thing—you can tell them how you got through it, and how you can work it out, and how you worked it out. You can try to make their trial . . . easier than what you have been through."

Attending to Spirit isn't easy, she says. But it's necessary.

"It gets hard a lot to keep your faith, because it is hard to deal with," Diamond says. "But you just got to pray about it. I do lose my faith sometimes, but I have family that helps me get through it."

When Diamond feels faith slipping or God seems distant, she prays for a stronger connection and stronger belief. She learned to pray from her oldest auntie, who taught her when she was a child. Now Diamond prays several times a day—silently when alone and out loud in person or over the phone with her aunties, grandmother, and church members.

Prayer reminds Diamond that God wants her to be a testimony to others—that her suffering has a purpose.

"God put everybody here for a reason," she says. "When he put you here for a reason, he want you to do it, because that shows a meaning in life. Everybody has their own feeling of what hope is, because people go through different things. . . . Some people let their illness get them down, like I do sometimes. They just seem depressed. They seem like they have a cloud over their head. But these [hopeful] kids, they do not let their illness get through; they talk to other people their age; they are very active, energetic—just, they feel good inside."

Diamond's story points toward consistent, positive religious coping: she works with God, connects to others, seeks divine love and care, feels communion with something beyond herself, and finds purpose in her experience. Her story also illustrates a hallmark result of attending to Spirit: turning inward, to access spiritual realities and resources, leads sick children outward again with an expanded perspective. In turning to Spirit, they tend also to slowly look beyond the treatment room and personal concerns to engage with the world and the concerns of others.

In the beginning of their illness, sick children focus on outer resources, seeking personal health and comfort from the people and activities around them. They strengthen their sense of agency and influence in relation to the treatment team and the illness. But as they experience the unpredictable and uncontrollable nature of illness, they realize their lives will never be "normal" in the ways they desire, no matter what they or others do. Human power cannot domesticate kidney disease, and this realization causes many children with chronic illness to seek spiritual power as an ally. Seeking consolation beyond the human, they grasp that Goodness loves and values them whether or not they're "normal" by their standards or the standards of the world. This insight turns them outward again with a new sense of compassion and empathy. They pivot beyond themselves and beyond the transplant clinic or dialysis unit to offer their gifts to the world by giving care and support to others. Purpose sustains hope, and children discover purpose in part by attending to Spirit.

"Because of the disease," fifteen-year-old Leo says, "you learn things to use to help other people who are sick."

. . . .

Leo's insight points toward the relational dimensions of chronic illness, the way sickness calls people out of themselves and into the world. Hope, for the children who talked with me, isn't a feeling or virtue or individual resource; it's a shared asset deeply entangled in connection to others, an ability to influence relationships, and a nascent awareness that Goodness expects them to participate in and contribute to the flourishing of others. I understand it this way: Attending to Spirit creates contemplative space, in which sick children can notice, identify, and claim how illness equips them to benefit others. By placing their own illness in a broader, transcendent context, they claim a sense of vocation shaped largely by the landscape of illness—a compassionate, altruistic commitment to easing the burden of sick people and of those who are temporarily well.

Learning to attend to Spirit is, itself, a product of relationships and altruistic commitments. Many sick children talk about a wisdom figure—a grandparent, aunt, pastor, hospital chaplain, or family friend, among others—who taught them faith and coached them in attending to Spirit. These are people present in the midst of illness not to attend to the details of treatment or pay the bills or worry about transportation but just to be with sick children—taking time to listen, to encourage, and to introduce children to Spirit in behavioral ways by teaching them to pray, to rely on scripture, to trust the goodness of the world. Wisdom figures offer guidance, presence, and consolation to children, usually through relationships that began long before diagnosis and the onset of chronic illness. They offer a perspective that models for sick children how to make positive, spiritual or religious, sense of pain and suffering. They help children understand faith as a partnership not only between people and God but also between people and people—and broader communities. Congregations and other spiritual communities mediate the consolation of Spirit by visiting children in the hospital, sending them gifts and cards, or emailing them to check in or offer encouragement. Wisdom figures matter because children initially trust Goodness because other, older people trust it too. Sick children trust their own ability to cope with illness because others voice confidence that children can cope with the help of God. In the end, children have faith not only in God but also in the people around them. Relationships with wisdom figures mirror, model, and create the faith and trust that children place in God.

I wonder if the transpersonal dimensions of hope also emphasize something about humanity: We are larger than our material, biological bodies, embedded in a matrix of relationships and energies that exceed awareness. These relationships and energies call us to a purpose beyond ourselves and bigger than our egos. We not only create identity, power, and meaning through action but also receive them from sources larger than our personalities and communities. Hope and humanity need imagination, intuition, and transcendent intimacy. Children seem more aware than grown-ups, sometimes, of the transpersonal aspects of hopefulness and of meaning that sustain human thoughts, actions, and relationships.

CHAPTER 5

CHOOSING TRUST

You should decide to have hope in yourself, because you know you are going to turn out okay. You have all these great people taking care of you, and they are here to help you.

—DESAREE, seventeen-year-old dialysis patient

Just stay strong and never give up, and that's enough.

—MAX, twelve-year-old dialysis patient

Enjoy life before you die.

—JAMES, seventeen-year-old transplant recipient

As we've seen, diagnosis sparks a crisis for children and their families; it scatters plans and priorities the way an autumn wind scatters fallen leaves. But new priorities emerge as children claim power, find community, and attend to spirit. Meanwhile, end-stage kidney disease, like any chronic illness, settles into a demanding but boring routine for children and their families: driving to and from dialysis, monitoring food and fluids, getting blood drawn, keeping track of medications, planning for fatigue and side effects. Temporary crises flare—a change in symptoms or unexpected surgery, for example—but coping mostly consists of maintaining patterns that seldom vary. As illness becomes an ordinary part of their lives, children finesse the sources of hope.

"I've learned a lot over these years," muses Nick, seventeen. He's sitting on an examination table at the transplant clinic. After years of treatment—diagnosed at five years old, both kidneys removed at thirteen, and more than two years of dialysis—he considers himself an expert on the ups and downs of the illness.

"I want to share with the rest of the children," he says. "I want to tell the children about me and what I went through. If I can relate to them, or if they can relate to me, I want to share my stories with them. That way, they can go through life not being—They don't have to be anxious, or they don't have to be scared about surgery. . . . I want to be able to share and tell them there is nothing to worry about. If they don't have hope, I want to give them hope and, if they do have hope, just give them more. So it's kind of a win-win situation."

This altruism—a desire to support other children living with kidney disease—runs through the practice of what I call choosing trust, especially among adolescents. Sick kids often talk about trust—trusting others, trusting treatment, trusting God—and as I conceptualize the theme, I find that trust involves positivity, gratitude, service, confidence, safety, and an awareness of death. Patients like Nick choose to trust what they have learned from (and because of) disease, even when their primary objects of hope—such as a successful transplant or a complete cure—do not materialize. In choosing trust, they integrate technical information from the medical team with an inner confidence about their well-being—a sort of spiritual assurance. Choosing trust leads children to turn outward and use their gifts, wisdom, and resources to benefit the world.

As a facet of hoping, choosing trust involves agency, relationships, and a growing recognition of internal resources. Children (like most people, in my experience) initially seem unaware of the pre-diagnosis resources and knowledge that help them sustain hope in the midst of kidney disease. Rather, they base their trust primarily in the interdisciplinary team's expertise. Their own values, and their confidence in a desirable, personal future, play a secondary role.

As a hopeful practice, choosing trust involves a positive attitude, confidence, gratitude, service to others, awareness of death, and a sense of safety; it can also have a spiritual dimension. Making a choice to trust seems to create confidence in a child's own ability to act. It relieves intra-psychic and spiritual suffering and generates possibilities. Choosing trust moves children beyond concern for their own well-being to a fertile desire to benefit the world. Finding ways to "give back" what they have received—especially, to activate a special, intuitive connection with caregivers and other chronically ill people—can be a significant part of making meaning of illness for some children. This type of generous altruism matters in the midst of chronic illness; renal patients who actively support friends and family are significantly less likely to die over the course of a year than those who simply receive support from others.[1]

This chapter illustrates how chronically ill children can, at times, return to the "normal" world with insights that benefit others. As a hopeful practice, trusting focuses on the horizontal and immanent dimensions of life, a shift from the vertical and transcendent focus of attending to spirit. Choosing trust reflects not only the personal and social resources that children bring to the experience of disease but also gifts received as a part of illness. It creates an active, enthusiastic stance toward life despite adversity, converting children's grief to desire—specifically, a yearning to reduce the world's pain and their suffering. Trust seems to lead to wisdom.

More than two-thirds of the children I interviewed talk about choosing trust as a dimension of hope. The same number emphasize attending to Spirit, but they talk about Spirit more often than trust. This suggests that children see choosing trust as less important than three other hopeful practices: realizing community, claiming power, and attending to Spirit. In addition, trust seems more important to girls (62 percent of those who talk about it) than to boys (38 percent) and to Black and Brown children of both sexes (81 percent) than to White children (19 percent).

I'm not sure how to interpret these differences, but I suspect they point toward the ways that the dominant culture in the United States and parts of Europe rewards boys and White children who value independence, self-sufficiency, mastery, and control over connection, communal resources, the commons, and the wisdom of others.[2] Might it be that White boys, especially, are taught to value, trust, and rely on themselves rather than a community or a greater good, to understand relationships as transactional and instrumental rather than as an essential part of their identity? If so, how could this shape their willingness and ability to choose trust?

POSITIVITY, GRATITUDE, MATURITY, AND LOVE

The stories children tell about hope suggest that intention matters. They weigh the evidence, judge the trustworthiness of the interdisciplinary team, assess their own abilities to influence the disease, and attend to the presence and consolation of Spirit; then they choose to trust that there are reasons to hope. The will—the capacity to choose and to make something happen—plays a big role in sustaining hope.

"I don't let pain or my disease take control over me," says fifteen-year-old Bradley, a dialysis patient. "I know there's something better; I know there's something else rather than just letting it come over me. . . . I just live day by day, year by year. I don't think about the now. I think about the future—how I can do stuff . . . how I can give back. . . . I *believe* there is hope."

Other children make similar choices, framing trust as a decision that can precede or inform other hopeful practices. "It's like you have, like, you trust something," says eleven-year-old Ryan, a transplant recipient. Children emphasize five types of experience when they talk about trust: positivity, gratitude, maturity, feeling loved, and finding purpose.

POSITIVITY

Nick insists that hope comes down to attitude: No matter what happens, he says, you simply choose to trust that good things such as receiving a kidney transplant will happen.

"It's a matter of how you feel," he says. "I mean, if you have a dead mind that says, 'Oh, this is never going to happen; I am just giving up,' then that is not the right attitude. But if you have the feeling that says, 'Oh well, one day it's going to happen; it's coming soon, I just have to be—I just have to wait. I will be patient. I will accept what I can change, and I just have to wait, and God is going to work his magic,' it is just going to happen one day, and one day you just get what you expect."

Thirteen-year-old Gina concurs. "It's what you set your mind to," she tells me. She's working on school assignments as she sits through dialysis. "Don't think of what the negatives would be, because if you think of the positives, you have a better chance— and if you think of the negatives, then normally nothing comes out right."

Children who emphasize positivity expect good things to happen. They tell each other not to take life for granted, to believe their health can improve. "Don't give up!" they say. "Have a great attitude! Trust that things will get better!"

These aren't empty, feel-good platitudes; they direct attention and prime the subconscious (perhaps unintentionally) to notice subtle improvements, hidden strengths, and moment-by-moment opportunities to shift attitudes and behaviors. Children use positive thoughts as mantras to turn their minds toward the attitudes that help them maintain hope, cope with suffering, and manage illness:

"Believe in yourself!"

"Be strong!"

"Be patient!"

"Have courage!"

I heard children recite these phrases over and over to themselves and to others in dialysis units and transplant clinics, similar to Tibetan monks using contemplative slogans—short phrases—to purify intentions, or athletes and business leaders using daily affirmations to set intentions. At first, I dismissed the words as "self-talk" or positive thinking. These phrases *are* self-talk, but they become something more, and over time I learned to see the repetition as a practice that develops the virtues of confidence, courage, patience, and strength in the midst of suffering. Eleven-year-old Brittany, a dialysis patient, puts it this way: "Hope is nothing but just believing in yourself."

Desaree, seventeen, says training her attitude helped her heal, even though she can't change the fact that she needs dialysis to survive.

"I am positive because I know it is helping me," she says. "I know it is keeping me healthy. . . . If I am pretty negative, it is just going to make me, like, embarrassed and sad about everything else. So, I will be positive, and that makes me happy and good."

GRATITUDE

Related to positivity, yet distinct from it, is the practice of gratitude. Being thankful seems to help children choose trust; by paying attention to what's going well and celebrating it, sick children increase their confidence that more good things—as yet unrecognized—are unfolding in the moment and approaching from the future. Children are experts at being grateful for small, specific things—not so much broad, global topics like

"I'm thankful for my family," but more granular awareness of good things in life: "I'm grateful for the way my mom cooks my favorite food on Sunday nights before dialysis." The children I talk with enjoy a breeze on a searing-hot day, notice the color of the sun shining through red tulips, savor the taste of Rocky Road ice cream (and the crunch of its almonds). They talk with gratitude about these types of daily encounters. Children know these small pleasures aren't permanent and not a certainty, nor do they erase physical or psychosocial suffering. But children with end-stage renal disease don't take good things for granted; they look for, name, and celebrate small wins and pleasures, including those experienced by others.

Children also express gratitude for their healthcare teams. They notice when a doctor, nurse, or phlebotomist acts with respect and kindness. A lab tech's positive attitude or goofy jokes can make them smile, and children reciprocate, joking with team members or offering kind words when someone seems to be having a tough day. They like it, too, when team members teach them about kidney disease and how to manage it, and they also appreciate team members who link patients at different stages of the disease to create opportunities for informal peer mentoring. Sick children give thanks for these small acts of kindness; they are especially grateful when team members help them notice, name, and respond to wisdom gleaned from chronic illness. "They are not just doing their job," says twelve-year-old Max, a transplant patient. "They are doing it out of their heart."

Team members who teach about medical procedures and coach the skills needed to live well with disease prompt children to gain "more maturity and more confidence," says fourteen-year-old Etta, a transplant recipient. "More maturity . . . because, like, you've been through, like, a lot, and you're more confident because you know, like, everything is going to be okay. . . . Give the patient all the information and all the guidance that they need for after the transplant and before the transplant. Tell them what to expect. . . . Give them the skills to do it. Yeah, give them the skills."

Eighteen-year-old Amy, a dialysis patient, was diagnosed with kidney disease at infancy. She remembers how the team provided information that relieved the terror she felt when she started dialysis.

"They told me how it worked and what it can do for me and stuff like that," she says, "the parts of the machine and what they do. They showed me some doll that had the dialysis catheter in it. When they explained it to me, it actually made me feel better; it did not seem as scary after they told me what they had to do and all that to put the catheter in. I guess it made me have more hope."

Children's gratitude extends far beyond the help they receive from the interdisciplinary team. They also recognize the good things that happen to others beyond their immediate circles.

Nick remembers waking up grouchy after surgery. His incisions hurt, the bed felt hard, and his head was woozy. He didn't feel like eating, and the people around him were irritating. His mother turned on the television to distract him.

"I saw this boy on the news," Nick remembers. "He had gotten a kidney transplant, and I was happy for him. . . . I was happier for him than I was for myself. . . . I was in a lot of pain, and seeing him on TV, playing with the doctor—that made me happy. In the midst of all that pain, I was happy."

Initially, I was surprised by how often sick children give thanks for the good things that happen to other people. I assumed, subconsciously, that illness drove children inward; I expected them to focus on their own health and concerns. But children in the dialysis unit and transplant clinic keep track of each other and what's happening in terms of friends, family, accomplishments, and illness. They encourage each other, cheer small wins, and show excitement when friends get good news.

Sick children not only suffer together; they also celebrate together, even when they don't know each other well.

This capacity for taking joy in the good fortune of others, the ability to celebrate good things beyond oneself, reminds me of the Buddhist virtue *mudita*, the satisfaction that comes from celebrating other people's well-being even when our own situations might be tragic. The presence of this virtue leads people to delight in the success and good fortune of others without feeling envious or greedy. Known as "sympathetic joy," mudita is often considered the most difficult virtue to cultivate. Yet taking joy in the joy of others, it's said, makes people more secure in their own happiness. Could it be that secure people find it easier to trust the world, themselves, and each other?

MATURITY, CONFIDENCE, CHOICE

As Etta noted, sick children gain maturity and confidence as they learn and understand how to care for themselves. They develop a certain determination or resolve that gives them the courage to choose trust. Many attribute their maturity to living with disease.

"We have to grow up a little more faster," says nineteen-year-old Devine, a dialysis patient. "We have to learn about, like, how hard it is to live. Other children, they don't necessarily get spoiled, but they don't have to go in that hospital. They don't have to study as hard to keep up in school. They don't have to do things twice as hard, like we do. I think children that grow up in [the] hospital or who go to the hospital a lot are a little bit more mature."

That maturity lends chronically ill children a quiet confidence. They rarely feel sorry for themselves; they accept illness and its limitations, and they know they're unlikely to live as long as healthy peers. They expect health setbacks, but they see improvements that follow a setback as a second chance to achieve their dreams. They're ready to move on once a difficulty passes. They don't linger on the bad stuff.

Nick, for example, doesn't dwell on his surgeries or his transplants, and he doesn't talk about them with others.

"I am fine," he says. "I am perfectly fine, and I walk around every day like I am fine. Just be. Just live it. Just do the things that you would normally do. If you just got surgery or something like that, and, like, you back to normal, you have no pain or anything like that, just act like you never got it; the surgery never happen at all. If somebody brings it up then, yes, you can discuss it. But don't let it get to you. I mean, it is over; you back to normal; you are 100 percent. Just finish whatever you were doing."

Children with this maturity or confidence talk about hope as voluntary, something they choose. They decide to hope, despite evidence for despair. They strive toward it with intention in ways that others can perceive as illogical, irrational, and unemotional. For sick children, hope is an option rather than a feeling. They persevere by choosing possibility, power, and joy. Emily, eleven, told me that kidney disease teaches her to keep going. "What I learned the most," she tells me, "is, it does not matter how many problems we will have or how many bad things you are thinking in your life. You should enjoy, because you are only going to live it once."

EXPERIENCING LOVE

A part of choosing trust, especially for girls, relates to the heart-felt presence of others. Children say being surrounded by family, friends, and competent caregivers reminds and assures them that they are loved. The meaning children give to the ways others care for them has clear connections to the hopeful practice of realizing connections. Knowing they are loved makes them feel safe; life seems less chaotic, and they sense more choice, more freedom, and more meaning in life. These elements make it easier to choose trust as a hopeful practice.

FINDING PURPOSE

Alongside positivity, gratitude, maturity, and love, children describe a fifth element of trust: finding purpose in the midst of illness. Sometimes, this is related to their practices of attending to Spirit; some children find direction and meaning in their understanding of what God or the Ultimate seeks to accomplish in their lives. Claiming a purpose—that is, having clarity about the positive meaning that their goals and values bring to suffering, treatment, relationships, and yearnings for "normal"—seems to solidify sick children's ability to choose trust. They believe that because of their illness, they will make a lasting difference in the world. They see themselves as part of something bigger, using purpose to construct a story about why their illness matters. This process creates meaning and sustains hope; in fact, having purpose is so important that researchers at the University of Wisconsin identify it as one of four pillars of a healthy mind (alongside awareness, connection, and insight).[3]

Some sick children say that living with kidney disease equips them to help others in unique ways. Older adolescents, especially, say they want to use their experiential knowledge to care for people with chronic illness and thus benefit the world—a common occurrence among patients with life-threatening illness.[4] Children make meaning of their illness in part by finding ways to "give back" what they have received and to activate a special spiritual or transpersonal connection to caregivers and other chronically ill patients.

Etta, fourteen, wants to become a nurse in part because she says she knows what it's like to have end-stage renal disease.

"Most of the nurses and doctors haven't been there," she says. "I just want to, like—If anybody has questions, then, yeah,

I'll answer them, because I have been there. Just saying, 'I know it hurts' and being truthful about it. I could say, 'I know what you're going through' and mean it, instead of just those doctors saying, 'I know it hurts' or whatever. I already went through it. They'll know somebody actually knows what they're going through, and they can have somebody to talk to.'"

Children describe two types of knowledge they gain from living with kidney disease. First, they internalize a pragmatic understanding of what it takes to stay healthy as they integrate medical information from the healthcare team with a spiritual assurance of their own well-being. Second, they develop an empathy or wisdom that allows them to connect with and understand suffering people. This seems to be the type of knowledge Etta emphasizes.

Children express this empathic wisdom in transpersonal terms and almost always in terms of career and vocation: as we've seen in previous chapters, many of the children I talked with want to become pediatric doctors or nurses. While remaining concerned about their own well-being, they expand toward an altruistic, generative focus on the well-being of others living with chronic illness. Inspired by gratitude for what they have learned from the healthcare team, they seek to give back to others.

Giving back emerges naturally as children choose trust; it's easier to have a sense of purpose when you trust caregivers, see the world as a safe place, and experience others responding to your needs. (The psychologist Erik Erikson understood this when he identified trust as a child's first developmental task and a necessary condition for hope.)[5] Claiming a purpose becomes a way of expressing trust in yourself, the world, the future, and the value of living with chronic illness. Purpose helps children deal with adversity; it is a key factor in recovering from a major trauma, and it is linked to better cognitive abilities, lowered risk of heart problems and stroke, deeper learning, greater persistence, and more effective self-regulation.[6] In addition, children with a sense of purpose do better in school, stay in school longer, earn more, and ultimately have higher net worth as adults.[7]

TRUST AS A GATEWAY TO VIRTUE

By now you've sensed that the five hopeful practices adopted by sick children (connection, power, Spirit, trust, and identity) aren't separate, sequential, or developmental. Children employ them simultaneously; the practices arise together, intermingling to influence, strengthen, and reinforce each other. It can be difficult to tell where one begins and another ends; often, it's the outcome that clarifies what practice a child has used in any given moment. The practice of choosing trust flows through the activities of realizing connections, claiming power, attending to Spirit, and maintaining identity. When trust leads children to claim embodied gifts, understandings, and purposes, for example, they are also maintaining identity (as described in chapter 6); when they turn outward in altruistic ways, incorporating the gifts of illness into their vision of life and sense of identity, they are also claiming power (chapter 3) and realizing connections (chapter 2) beyond the world of end-stage renal disease. The sense of support and safety children solidify by attending to Spirit (chapter 4) helps them choose trust, and engaging trust's five elements—positivity, gratitude, maturity, love, and purpose—can become concrete ways of appreciating and manifesting abundance in the midst of painful realities.

Children choose trust in large part because it relieves immediate spiritual, psychosocial, and existential suffering by placing sickness in a larger frame of meaning. It gives them some control over their experience of illness; no matter what, they can choose a positive attitude, express gratitude, exercise choice, and remember they are loved. Choosing trust also generates possibilities for a future in which children see themselves not as "sick kids" but as wise companions with a purpose. As such, they imagine using knowledge and skills gained by living through diagnosis and treatment to do good in the world—not despite illness but in part because of it. They are motivated to some degree by a yearning for the happiness and wholeness of others—a shift toward a "desire for the wellbeing of all beings . . . [a] conscious connection with all life," which activists Joanna Macy and Chris Johnstone see as evidence of an awakened heart-mind.[8] Choosing trust often indicates that children see themselves as offering value to the broader community. It signals that they are venturing forth from illness to contribute to the "normal" world; as such, the practice entails a shift outward, a return to the horizontal and immanent dimensions of hope after the primarily vertical and transcendent focus of attending to Spirit.

The children who talk with me suggest that the practice of choosing trust manifests through relationships. They *learn* to choose trust; it doesn't just happen. Two elements seem to contribute. First, consistent and dependable caregivers convince sick children that they are safe and secure despite illness; suffering does not and cannot overwhelm or erase them. Children feel and act confident and brave because they believe the people and organizations in their lives will be there if they fail or need help. Second, parents, healthcare workers, teachers, and peers coach sick children into a trusting stance. This occurs through repeated, gentle reminders to stay positive and via questions that encourage dreaming and contributions to the family, the healthcare process, the community, and the world. These interactions gradually shape a trusting stance that children internalize. They believe that their reality exceeds the influence of illness; interrupted plans, social isolation, and pain aren't the whole story. In response, children clarify their values and reprioritize their desires to acknowledge and address this larger context.

The ways that community creates the conditions for choosing trust go beyond developmental and psychosocial contributions.

Yes, choosing trust requires secure attachment and existential confidence—a sense that the world and caregivers are dependable, consistent, available, safe, supportive, and responsive. But choosing trust also requires that children feel confident in material, sociopolitical conditions that reduce fear and challenge scarcity—housing, transportation, education, income, and community; sufficient, affordable healthcare; well-trained doctors, nurses, and medical professionals; access to medication; affordable insurance; freedom from violence; and more. When communities attend to these material needs in ways that allow children to choose trust with confidence, children receive what Buddhist traditions call the gift of fearlessness (*abhayadana*), a result of the "practice of creating secure conditions for the vulnerable in order to protect their lives and to relieve their fear."[9] When the community provides protection, resources, stability, peace, and other support, children can flourish free from the fear that scarcity or danger threatens their lives. A child's ability to hope depends as much on material and sociopolitical realities as on psychosocial and spiritual experiences. The outer conditions precede and sustain the inner virtue and personal practices of hope.

When children choose trust, when they are no longer caged by fear or constrained by the demands of kidney disease, they develop a new confidence. When they step into a situation, they lead with the elements of trust, and the stance becomes a dimension of their identity outside the hospital, clinic, and treatment room—a virtue that they practice and value rather than a pragmatic coping strategy. As such, it emerges from and creates a sense of stability. They see their world as safe, consistent, and dependable, even when life suggests otherwise, which allows them to have courage even when pain seems in charge. Trust transforms the pain, shame, and doubt that can accompany chronic illness, transmuting them into confidence, purpose, and wisdom. In short, trust redefines "normal." Sick children who choose trust no longer expect to escape finitude, fix illness, or get rid of pain, but to be present with others in the midst of it all. They know that illness and suffering are part of "normal," not a stain that places them outside community.

Yet it's naive to think that choosing trust erases the suffering associated with chronic illness and cements a child's hope, forever and ever, amen. Suffering continues to threaten a child's sense of self, no matter how positive or trusting the child's stance toward disease, illness, and the capacity for improvement. Finding ways to maintain identity against the disease's erosion of self becomes a final hopeful practice in the midst of chronic illness.

CHAPTER 6

MAINTAINING IDENTITY

*Always have hope; hope is a beautiful word—telling
me to go forward, complete my dreams, be who I am.*

—SMILEY, fifteen-year-old dialysis patient

*The way to find hope is through people, through
yourself and the people who really care for you. . . .
They are the ones who keep pushing you to do things
that you don't want to do, and they keep pushing you
to do the things you want to, because they care for
you, and they want what is best for you.*

—ANDREW, eighteen-year-old transplant recipient

Kidney disease slowly erodes young people's identities, eating
away at everything that defined them prior to diagnosis.
It distorts bodies; steals time from friends, sports, and school;
restricts activities; changes family routines and relationships;
strains finances; and shifts family priorities as disposable income decreases. Money previously available for travel, sports,
and recreation must be allocated to disease management. These
indignities warp every part of life—physical, social, emotional,
spiritual, relational, communal, and systemic—and the losses
can happen faster than a child's ability to make sense of what's

happening. How do sick children sustain a sense of self when disease threatens every part of identity?

Two months ago, Velma was a vivacious sixteen-year-old with long, shiny black hair and honey-colored skin. A few days before spring break, her eyes got puffy. Then her blood pressure rocketed. Her family took her to the ER, and she was admitted to the hospital, where doctors biopsied her kidney. Later that day, she started dialysis. For two weeks, she lay in a hospital bed far from home while the treatment team worked to stabilize her kidneys. Now she gets dialysis three days a week, recovering at home between treatments. Medications make her hair patchy and her skin itchy and flaky. Her clothes no longer fit, hanging off her hips and shoulders, and she feels lonely a lot of the time.

"I don't go to school. I have to get homeschooled, so I don't see my friends," Velma says. "My family comes and visits me, but, like, it changed me—like, my body. I lost a lot of weight, and it makes my hair fall out and little things like that. I like the fact that I lost weight; that was, like, the best part. But sometimes I think I am going to go bald. And then, also, like, I cannot do a lot of things. Like, I cannot go swimming and do, like, other stuff, like take a normal shower."

As the ravages of kidney disease collide with the stormy realities of puberty and adolescence, sick children struggle to identify the parts of themselves unchanged by disease. Yet they are also discovering and constructing themselves as sexual, gendered, and independent people. They learn that their interests and beliefs differ from those of family and elementary school friends, even as social isolation and physical limitations make it difficult to engage typical teenage exploration and develop new relationships. Chronic illness can complicate the exploration of values, relationships, and commitments necessary to develop a strong sense of self during the transition toward young adulthood.

REMEMBERING "NORMAL"

Children with end-stage renal disease always know they're different from healthy peers. Emily, eleven, turns down invitations to sleepovers because she has to be in bed, prepped for dialysis, and connected to the cycler by 7 p.m. Ten-year-old Jake hates his restricted diet, and he hates that during dialysis, he's required to keep his arms and legs straight, with his head lower than his feet—a position that not only gives him a headache but, worse, makes it impossible to play video games. Ebony, fourteen, can't eat the cafeteria food at school, which makes her self-conscious with friends at lunch; Trafford, seventeen, is permitted a single French fry each week, which cramps his style when he's out with buddies. Eighteen-year-old Striker plunged into depression when his dad lost a job and left the family without health insurance, delaying the transplant Striker counted on before his senior year. Enrique, fifteen, no longer plays football, and Leo, also fifteen, quit playing goalie in soccer because of the tube that sticks out of his abdomen like a spigot.

"It is kind of sad, because you are not like other kids," says Brittany, the eleven-year-old who receives dialysis. "I kind of feel sad at times because I am not like other kids. I cannot run around and play in gym, and . . . you know . . ." Her words trickle off. Brittany's school held a fundraiser for her medical expenses, which made her grateful but also embarrassed. Her classmates didn't need financial help.

Even Riley—the positive, eager fourteen-year-old with a guardian angel, the girl spunky enough to search Facebook for a donated kidney—gets overwhelmed.

"You have those moments when you are just, like, I am sick of this," she says. "I just want to stop everything. Why did this have to happen? I am just, like, completely . . ." She sighs. "Like, I am done with this."

Young people with kidney disease say their bodies remind them daily that they're different from other kids. Finding ways to maintain pre-disease identities—athlete, pizza lover, risk-taker, gamer—becomes a way to sustain hope when collective losses threaten a child's self-image. Children with end-stage renal disease treasure people and activities that remind them who they were before diagnosis and treatment. Sports, friends, and family seem especially important.

As a means of sustaining hope, maintaining identity seems less critical than other strategies; slightly more than half of our research partners talk about it, especially boys. They invoke it far less often than trust, Spirit, power, and connection. But questions of identity become more salient as children age, and older adolescents in particular find maintaining identity a useful practice even as they learn new things about themselves and grow beyond their childhood sense of self. As a means of sustaining hope, maintaining identity seems primarily performative and agential—that is, something focused on what sick young people can still do, or do anew, despite limitations created by disease and its treatment that becomes true by taking action. Maintaining identity isn't something children believe but something they act on in small ways. As with choosing trust, maintaining identity emphasizes the immanent and horizontal dimensions of life. It draws primarily on resources children bring to the experience of illness but incorporates those developed during treatment—especially the ability to claim power and the wisdom of choosing trust.

When thirteen-year-old Gina was diagnosed, she didn't expect kidney disease to interrupt her life.

"I thought with all of this, you know, in ten or twelve years, I would still have to be taking medication or extra medication," she says. "Instead, they had to come out with dialysis. Then I had to have a tube put in. So then I didn't have much hope. Then my parents were like, 'Oh, no. You'll get better. You are going to be able to go out and play and hang out with friends. Don't just focus on that one little thing.' Then I will be able to have most of my normal life, just to be able not to be getting hooked up [to dialysis] every night. Then I could, like, stay over at a friend's house and stuff. Be a normal teenager."

The desire to be "normal" (or "more normal," in fourteen-year-old Etta's memorable phrase) shapes children's efforts to maintain identity. In chapter 3, I suggested that "normal" functions for sick children as shorthand for a preferred future, a state of well-being and wholeness that's always out of reach but motivates them to claim power. The practice of maintaining identity sharpens that vision: Sick children seek a future that *incorporates and builds on past identities*. When they invoke "normal," they point toward the life and self they knew before diagnosis—signaling, in part, a desire to reclaim a positive and resourceful past. It's difficult to know whether (temporarily) healthy adolescents are less concerned with past identities and more open to new ones, but it's clear that end-stage renal disease makes the usual challenges of identity formation more complex. Young people with end-stage renal disease try to preserve and carry forward the self that existed before they entered the territory of illness. Some also discover positive, new facets of identity as they cope with the disease. The practice of maintaining identity can include efforts to integrate these gifts and discoveries into post-disease life.

Two themes shape efforts to maintain identity: routines and relationships.

ROUTINES AND RELATIONSHIPS: ANCHORING IDENTITY

When I ask sick children what helps them hold on to their identity after diagnosis, the stories they tell are usually mundane. They talk about family dinners, gaming with friends, softball practice, and holiday traditions. They emphasize the rhythms and routines that shaped their lives before illness—consistent, ordinary moments they could count on. This doesn't surprise me; our sense of self relies on commonplace, even humdrum, activities in which we construct and receive our identity.

In the midst of chronic illness, the usual family routines— game night, grocery shopping, daily chores, taking out the garbage—remind sick children that they're more than patients, that disease can't steal their identities as sons, daughters, sisters, brothers, grandchildren, and cousins. Parents and grandparents set goals, offer encouragement, and help keep friends and extended family close. Sports practice, parties, video games, and social media keep young people in touch with peers. Children want daily life to assimilate illness, fitting it into what already exists, rather than restructuring everything around disease. What does this assimilation look like?

Sixteen-year-old Gared says his week has dialysis days and soccer days. Tuesday and Thursday, he goes to practice; Monday, Wednesday, and Friday, he goes to dialysis. Soccer days, he says, are real life; dialysis days give him a chance to rest.

Brittany, eleven, makes hanging out with friends a weekly priority. She says they keep her healthy by helping her exercise. On her own, she's afraid to try new things; she worries that she'll get hurt or damage the dialysis port in her chest. Not even her mom can coax her into taking risks. But her friends give her courage.

"I can trust them," she says. "They are always with me; they are with me through everything. They are true. It is kind of like, I can believe in some form—like, I can try and do anything around them. I would try and run or jump around like them, how they really do it. I feel safe around them because if I fall or anything, they are there to catch me."

On Sundays, fifteen-year-old Enrique insists on joining his cousins at church to lead a preschool class. No matter how bad he feels, he keeps his commitment. He teaches little kids to play H-O-R-S-E at the basketball hoop on the asphalt parking lot, helps them paint with watercolors and acrylics, and supervises their turns on the teeter-totter, swing set, and slide. As he does, his fatigue and loneliness go away. After church there's sometimes a party, a fundraiser, or another special event. Enrique stays for those. He goes home happy at the end of the day.

"My friends are there, and my cousins, so I don't think about the kidney," he says. "I don't think about, 'I have kidney disease.' I am just over there having fun. Like, I forgot my feeling that my kidneys were failing. It keeps me going—feeling like you are just normal, and you don't have any diseases."

Spending a day at church, woven into the community, keeps Enrique in touch with his identity as an athlete, a friend, a mentor, a volunteer, and a Christian. Kidney disease is just part of the routine.

While maintaining identity can focus on routines and relationships that were important before diagnosis, it also involves relationships developed *because* of treatment. Friends made during dialysis and at kidney camp (described in chapter 2), along with members of the healthcare team, shape who sick young people are now and who they're evolving into over time.

Desaree, seventeen, chats daily via text with a group of friends she met during dialysis. "We understand each other. Our problems are a little different—they are not the same—but . . . they have been there. They are the ones who has to deal with it; they are the ones who has to go through all that. They just know how it feels to be on dialysis. . . . You are not the same as everybody else, but in here"—she sweeps an arm around the dialysis unit—"we are all the same."

William, fifteen, delights in kidney camp for similar reasons.

"It is kind of a relief when you are around people . . . [and] everybody has the same thing," he says. "It is not that they can't make fun of each other; it is just like they don't bother to make fun of each other because it is not funny. . . . They think I am the same, a normal kid. . . . They don't sit and stare at you and point and laugh and whisper to each other about you. They just ask you when you started dialysis, how long you had been on dialysis. Sometimes they show each other scars or [ask] about what point that they go through and how they got started on dialysis, when they got the transplant and how long they had it."

For Enrique, the nurses matter a lot. They challenge him to think about the future. "They encourage me to get my grades up, and sometimes they just tell me to do good work at school so I could be better—a better life in the future and better work," he says. "They encourage me. They help me stay focused on my school and grades and all that. They actually care; they want me to have, like, a better life so that when I grow, I could pay for my medicines and all that—if I have a good job, I can get and pay for medicines and the future and all."

The interdisciplinary treatment team plays a particular role in maintaining identity.

RE-MEMBERING AND THE INTERDISCIPLINARY TEAM

It's Monday morning, and nineteen-year-old Jewell laughs with the nurses as they hook her up to the dialysis machine.

"So you think that boy likes you?" one nurse says, winking. Jewell grins.

"What else'd you do this weekend?" another nurse asks as he slips a needle into Jewell's catheter.

"Just went to the mall, hung out with my friends," Jewell says. "The usual."

"Tell me about those friends," says the nurse. "Those girls you play video games with."

Jewell launches into stories about each of her friends, swiping through photos on her phone to show the outfits they tried on at various stores.

Across the room another nurse asks fourteen-year-old Rob, "How'd you do on your test last week? And what happened to your brother—did he get in trouble like you thought he would?" They laugh as Rob tells a raucous story about his oldest sibling coming home after curfew to find their mom waiting.

These casual conversations relieve the tedium of treatment. But they also play a significant role in maintaining identity. The children I talk with emphasize that hope is nurtured by the ways that nurses, doctors, and other members of the interdisciplinary team ask informally about friends, family, school, vacation, and weekend activities. These conversations don't focus on gathering information for medical purposes but on creating and sustaining relationships and day-to-day living in the community of the dialysis unit and transplant clinic.

Healthcare workers who ask patients about their lives beyond the dialysis unit, remember the names of family members, and track worries and celebrations not only build relationships that make connections for the purpose of care; they also remind sick children of family and community identities unrelated to illness. Such questions communicate care and interest, and they acknowledge that there's more to children's lives than catheters, blood draws, urine output, and clinic visits. These conversations help children rehearse who they are, highlighting and strengthening the identities they constructed prior to diagnosis.

This type of re-membering—strengthening children's connections to the communities in which they are members—requires curiosity to help children identify and enrich relationships with the people who become cheerleaders and consultants in the midst of illness, people who create a circle of influence by being supportive, wise, and providing and eliciting resources for positive change.[1] Re-membering conversations contribute at least two hopeful strategies to young people with illness. First, they distract children from the immediate medical context, refocusing them on their identities and daily lives apart from disease. Second, they communicate the healthcare team's belief that a child has a present and future that include but are broader than the disease.

Both effects, children say, help them maintain their pre-disease identities and integrate dimensions of themselves that emerge through illness.

CARRYING FORWARD

Seeking to maintain identity—particularly those aspects valued before diagnosis—can, in some cases, indicate that young people with chronic illness (or perhaps their families) cling to a past that has changed rather than accepting the ways disease shapes their current lives. More often, I think, sick children aren't clinging to past identities but seeking to bring those identities into the future. Carrying pre-disease identities forward allows them to maintain consistency and gives meaning in the midst of illness. Earlier life stages continue "to be present, not lost, not left behind," as anthropologist Mary Catherine Bateson reminds us.[2] Re-membering who they have been and carrying new dimensions of identity into the future allow children to make commitments to themselves, their families, and their communities to care for their health—their "physical, mental, and social well-being"—for the sake of continuing to engage in activities and relationships they value and of caring for those who experience similar challenges.[3] This becomes a dimension of "normal" grasped and sustained because of illness.

"You live what you wanted to live," says seventeen-year-old Trafford, a transplant recipient. "Like, live the life now that you wanted to before. Once you get a kidney transplant, you will be able to live what you wanted . . . , kind of like before. Live all the days. Live long. Like, do what you want to do, like stuff like that. Basically, it is just keep going and move forward. Just keep moving forward."

Sustaining hope by knowing who you have been and who (and what) you want to carry from the territory of illness allows some sick children to dwell creatively in the world. They feel anchored, certain of themselves, at home no matter what's happening.

"You feel comfortable—comfortable anywhere," says Gareth, a sixteen-year-old dialysis patient. "I mean here [in the dialysis unit], at home, at hospital, at doctor—anywhere. . . . Just have hope in yourself."

CHAPTER 7

LEARNING FROM CHILDREN

The time I spent with children in the dialysis unit and transplant clinic reshaped my experiences of hope. As I've said throughout the book, I learned more than expected while listening to them, sitting beside them during treatment, and observing clinic appointments. But my more significant learning—larger, subtler, and perhaps more enduring—happened as I sat with their words over time. For several years, I read and reread the transcripts of our conversations, comparing what one child said to the stories of others. As I understood and internalized their perspectives, my questions about hope grew more subtle. I wondered if I'd ever known as much as they did about sustaining hope in the midst of adversity. When I wrote or spoke about hope, I'd ask myself: "Would Nick agree? What would Etta say? Am I being honest enough to make Diamond grin and say, 'Amen!'?" The children in the study became mentors and companions as I continued to seek meaning and insight from their stories.

Gradually, the ideas that I brought to the research—that hope was an individual experience, focused on the future, related to feelings, and rooted in executive functioning skills—began to seem simplistic and perhaps naive. Receiving a cancer diagnosis in 2017 created a new gateway to the territory of illness, and I started testing what children told me in light of a threat to my life. I thought about how to make real connections with professionals, survivors, and patients during chemotherapy. I identified how I could appropriately claim power in relation to lymphoma. I explored different ways of attending to Spirit in the midst of illness, both during chemotherapy sessions and during the three weeks between treatments. I chose again and again to trust my doctors and nurses, my body, and my family. And as much as possible, I kept at the professional and personal activities that are central to my identity, even when I felt like crap: exhausted, nauseated, headachy, pale; bald, out of breath, and aching with bone pain as my body labored to produce white blood cells.

I discovered that engaging the practices I learned from children reoriented my attention to the present. I hoped for a cure, of course, and on some days barely kept afloat in an ocean of anxiety and worry, imagining how I'd spend my final months and years if treatment didn't work. (But it did! I have been cancer-free since 2017, officially in remission since 2022.) But the practices of hopeful children redirected me from imaginary futures, positive and negative, to notice and nurture the goodness saturating every day—even the bad ones. By purposely engaging community, power, Spirit, trust, and identity, I coped better with illness and the limitations I encountered. It was easier to choose hope, and the practices kept me realistic, anchored to facts and experiences, rather than caught up in fear and ungrounded optimism.

Over time, I let go of the idea that I could analyze and systematize children's words (and my own experience) into an overarching theory that explains and predicts hope. Would that even be useful? These days, I feel certain that we can't capture or tame "hope." It emerges on its own terms, a creative, radiant, fluid energy that discloses—briefly—the hidden abundance of our lives. We don't so much create hope or offer it to each other as track it through the landscape of experience. Sometimes we recognize or discover hope between yearning and grief, but it remains indescribable, even in the moment. We can't hold it in our hands or save it for later, but we can help each other notice when it comes near.

The fact that hope among chronically ill children belongs to the present rather than the future might be the biggest takeaway from my learning. Hope begins as a social resource before children internalize it as a personal resource, and it has strong relational dimensions. It emerges from interactions with caregivers, families, and friends, and it creates a critical vision of what is possible. That vision helps children clarify who and how they want to be in the midst of chronic illness. Hope isn't a static, universal construct; it varies by sex, race, ethnicity, timelines, and socioeconomic realities. What children know about hope invites us to revise healthcare practices, psychological models, and spiritualities that focus on hope as an emotion, a virtue, and a future-oriented reality. It offers lessons for the broader experience of chronic illness and for the role of hope beyond healthcare crises. Those lessons include the priority of community in maintaining hope; the roles of mutuality, vulnerability, and connection in establishing trust in healthcare; the vibrancy of spiritual disciplines as a gateway to the transfinite dimensions of hope; the need for shared power across difference; the potency of shifting one's relationship to disease; and the need to revise theories of hope oriented toward the future and ultimacy to affirm instead that hope is local, related to the present, and oriented primarily toward place and community and only secondarily toward time.

Children diagnosed with end-stage renal disease bring to treatment a variety of relationships, emotional habits, family traditions, faith understandings, and personal identities. They and their families enter the foreign territory of disease as sojourners, resident aliens who will dwell in that land for quite some time. The culture is strange; it threatens identities and creates a sense of loss that elicits lament. But they pitch their tents in the midst of a community already wise in the ways of the landscape and the culture of the disease, and it teaches them how to survive the territory. Its members do not expect children to give up the identities or traditions of their original places but instead expect them to value those dimensions of the child as gifts to the community.

Three questions guided me as I wrote the book: What do children know about being human that most grown-ups have forgotten? How do children's experiences reveal the limitations and distortions created by prevailing ideas about hope? How can we cultivate and nurture together our capacity to hope when despair seems rational? My responses to these questions weave throughout the chapters, and each chapter points toward possible ways to answer such questions in relation to the highlighted practice. Readers, no doubt, have their own sense of what these children's voices teach about the nature of humanity, how to broaden their own thinking about hope, and actions they can take to nurture hoping among the people they know and love. Here, in the final chapter, I want to briefly articulate what has stayed with me as I look back across the landscape of children's hope in the territory of chronic illness.

WHAT DO SICK CHILDREN KNOW ABOUT BEING HUMAN?

What sick children say about hope reminds me of five human realities I can usually downplay, ignore, or pretend don't exist due to my status and resources as a White, middle-aged, middle-class professional in the industrialized Global North. Grown-ups don't forget these realities, necessarily, but too often they don't make them a priority or treat them with appropriate respect.

First, health is temporary. Illness is a human norm. Sick children eventually accept that being unwell is natural; they don't expect to fix illness, escape pain, or transcend their limits, but they do expect to live well in their midst. Young people with kidney disease know that illness and suffering are normal, expected parts of life; eventually, everyone shares the experience, some more acutely and for longer periods than others. Rather than fighting illness and the limitations it creates, sick children incorporate them into their vision of what it means to be human. A life without sickness isn't life in its fullness, and accepting that can reduce our suffering when we (or those we love) become ill or lose abilities.

Second, humans live in a matrix of relationships and energies that exceed their biological bodies, and those relationships call us to purposes beyond ourselves. Sick children remind me that humans—all of us together and each of us as unique beings—belong to something bigger than our egos, our families, our communities, and our planet. No matter how much tragedy and evil we encounter, we can trust the goodness of that larger reality, and we can and must add to goodness in the places we live and move and have our beings. We don't have to be heroic or make grand gestures; sometimes our contributions to the good are tiny—being kind to a rude person, distracting a frightened child, teaching someone to breathe deeply when they're anxious. Sick children know that suffering people need partners rather than caregivers, that the nature and quality of our interactions matter more than our "official" roles and functions. We are here for each other, and hope emerges from our ability to connect meaningfully with others in the present moment.

Third, "health" depends on a person's relationship with the limits imposed by illness. It's not the (temporary) absence of disease that qualifies someone as healthy but their responses to the ways illness curtails freedom, independence, and functioning. If having limitations is a natural part of being human, how do we negotiate, navigate, and value the experiences of limits? At their best, chronically ill children don't treat their disease as an adversary; they understand it as a source of pain, wisdom, compassion, and maturity. People with chronic illness suffer, but suffering isn't the end of their stories; they also receive gifts, strength, and capacities from illness, resources they haven't encountered in other parts of life. In particular, they've found ways to endure, love, grow, and thrive in the absence of the "health" they desire. They live with suffering rather than struggling to escape it. We cannot sufficiently account for wholeness if we only consider abilities, what we and others can do.[1]

Fourth, the natural state of humanity is dependency, not autonomy. When we teach each other that our fundamental value depends on our ability to do things for ourselves, to function independently, to produce and consume as autonomous agents, we distort what it means to be human. Grown-ups should prioritize children's relational, emotional, and spiritual capacities over cognitive abilities, economic contributions, and potential participation in the workplace. Chronic illness shows children that dependency enriches their lives. While their own resources (or those of their families) might be limited, they're usually connected to someone(s) who can provide what they need. We strengthen children when we introduce them to communities and institutions and teach them to access the resources available beyond their families. Theologian David H. Jensen argues that children were created to live in a state of "graced vulnerability," needing relationships to thrive.[2] My time with sick children makes me believe that vulnerable children who are received with mutuality and equipped to be appropriately responsible can receive hope in and through communities of care that create outposts of abundance in the present moment.

Finally, humans can experience health in the midst of illness. We can realize our potential, reduce stress, work fruitfully, and contribute to the community without being cured. Rather than seeking victory over disease, we generate health by creating pragmatic solutions to the ongoing challenges of chronic illness and by promoting authentic relationships, spiritual engagement, and meaning-making, and by valuing each person's contribution to goodness and mutual flourishing. Health doesn't erase or remove the limitations created by illness; it integrates them into all dimensions of life and shares the resources necessary to thrive while living with disease.

HOW DO SICK CHILDREN EXPAND UNDERSTANDINGS OF HOPE?

Throughout the book, I've suggested that hope among sick children has existential, sociocultural, and material dimensions. It involves both the resources they bring to the experience of disease and the relational and psychosocial gifts they receive as a result of illness. Children convince me that we must imagine, perceive, and enact hope in ways that move beyond the prevailing emphases on emotion, cognition, and virtue. I also suspect we need simpler ways of conceptualizing hope. Psychologists, for example, distinguish between global hope (a disposition), domain-specific hope (that is, hope related to specific areas of life, such as school, athletics, relationships, or work), and goal-specific hope (about a specific desired outcome). But sick children don't have such specific, granular ways of thinking about hope; for them, hope manifests as a single reality experienced at particular moments, usually through bonds shared with parents, caregivers, peers, family, and a transcendent reality.

Children's stories of hope suggest it doesn't happen "inside" people but between them. It can involve visions of the future but primarily attends to the present, the possibilities available to suffering people day-to-day. Children's hope turns them toward actions that honor and amplify Goodness, yet it's less about "right" or "beneficial" behavior than about a trusting, receptive stance toward the world. It entails carrying the past forward as well as constructing new realities in the future. For young people living with chronic illness, hope surfaces through the energy that leads us toward preferred futures; they do not hope in those futures but rather maintain hoping through the people and activities that help make those futures real. Hoping is a process, not a goal or an outcome.

The ways that children with chronic illness talk about hope help unmask the ways that prevailing, grown-up models of hope are individualistic, optimistic, temporal, patriarchal, Western, and neoliberal. Grown-up models can unintentionally promote stereotypically "masculine" characteristics—things like independence, risk-taking, self-sufficiency, assertiveness, confidence, and decisiveness—by socializing children into particular ways of thinking about and performing hope. Existing models of hope don't sufficiently attend to the moral, relational, and spiritual dimensions of hope, which puts those models at risk of becoming tools for exploitation. They can be (and are) co-opted to promote consumerist-consumptionist ideologies that colonize dreams, distort identities, and fail to challenge the status quo.

We need a spiritual, communal, relational, and collaborative model of hope appropriate to the developmental skills and abilities of children and youth. It should acknowledge hope's own agency in human lives, emphasizing that it doesn't depend on human abilities. It should attend to material and sociopolitical influences on hopefulness. It should encourage holistic engagement rather than a competitive, goal-centered stance; acknowledge relational connections and the ways that we depend on each other and creation; it should encourage modest confidence and caring respect; and it must treat hope as contextual rather than universal and independent.

HOW CAN WE CULTIVATE AND NURTURE HOPE TOGETHER?

In the midst of chronic illness, children's hopes are relational, active, transpersonal, and formative. They challenge dominant stories about what it means to be hopeful and what it means to be a child. This is a good thing, because our qualitative understandings of hope—what we believe about it, how it shapes our vision, and why we think it matters—tend to be dictated by culture and the sociopolitical and socioeconomic systems that mold our lives. (It's always wise to ask yourself, "Whose interests are served by this understanding?" when you find yourself thinking and acting in particular ways about hope—what it is, how it comes into being, what makes it legitimate.) Children's stories of hope in the midst of chronic illness convince me that its nurture and formation can be a liberative activity, a contribution to practices of freedom that relieve suffering and promote abundant life. Therefore, one of the most important ways we can cultivate hope together is by creating a normative vision of appropriate hope and teaching it to children.

Before I talk more explicitly about ways to promote hope together, however, I want to highlight the value of exploring hope in the context of chronic illness. Nurturing and sustaining hope in the midst of disease, identifying and intentionally practicing hopeful activities, help create and maintain well-being. Hope and hoping clarify identity, contribute to meaning-making, improve health outcomes, enhance coping, strengthen relationships, and help children manage illness effectively. They strengthen connections to groups and communities, increase competency and capabilities, and solidify a child's sense of self-worth. Yet attending to hope shapes children's lives beyond chronic illness as well.

Researchers tell us that hopeful children live more satisfying and meaningful lives in general, with or without disease. Learning about the relationship between hope and chronic illness in children provides wisdom about living with other types of suffering, resiliency, loss, and joy. Because all people experience losses, crises, and challenges, we can learn from those with chronic illness, who constantly "struggle with putting their lives together after disruptions, controlling time, creating continuity with past selves, reconstructing new selves, devising timemarkers [sic], noting turning points, and locating themselves in the past, present, or future."³ We see how they cope and thereby learn to respond more effectively to our own setbacks.

What sick children understand about hope, then, has implications for what it means to be a hoping human in general, regardless of age. For me, this realization became increasingly important as the global climate crisis began to dominate the world's imagination and a pandemic literally stopped the human world—interrupted "normal"—for years. These situations not only demand action but also present barriers to hope similar to those inherent in chronic illness. I began to wonder how humans can hope together in an environmentally uncertain world. How can we sustain hope when the planet's dis-ease truncates the future and seems to offer little opportunity for change big enough to repair the damage done to (and by) our collective body? Living in this broader social and historical moment shapes my understanding of children's hope because the experiences of chronic illness—disorientation, unpredictability, a sense of impending disaster, a shortened and limited future, and so forth—reflect in a microcosm the global experiences of people living in climate crisis. These days, all of humanity faces an uncertain and limited future—or, if not limited, at least significantly different from what we perceive as "normal." This ambiguous future intrudes on our lives and demands resiliency. Might it be possible that by paying attention to how children nurture hope in the midst of chronic illness, we can identify ways to strengthen the human response to climate crises, healthcare pandemics, and rising totalitarianism around the globe? Can practices of hope help orient us in a changing world?

Nurturing hope happens at multiple levels simultaneously. We nurture hope among individuals, families, and communities; through institutions that address the common good, including the legal system and public policies; through economic systems that ensure every child can access the resources they need to flourish; by caring for the cosmos; and by cultivating cultural stories, values, and habits that orient human activity toward particular relational, collaborative, communal and transpersonal activities by which specific hopes enter the world. As theologian Marlene Ferreras writes, "'Hope' is a reality revealed *in* the struggle," and we identify it by asking "who is present, what is happening, and what is taking place. . . . The question is never about when the future will arrive, for the future is continually emerging."[4]

We collectively strengthen community and power by engaging in grassroots activism that helps children and their families establish strong connections to social, civic, and educational organizations that can help them access resources they do not find in themselves or their immediate networks. We work to ensure that parents and families are not isolated but are connected to schools, businesses, and neighborhoods. In healthcare, we make patients partners in treatment rather than objects of care. We attend to Spirit and create trust by establishing personal, long-term relationships with children, teaching them the spiritual practices we use to stay connected to transcendent and transpersonal realities.[5] We introduce them to their ancestors and help children express their own spiritualities in the world. We show children the people and organizations working for the common good and talk about how our own values intersect with their activities. We attend to identity by helping each other clarify values and preferences, locate their sources, and bring them with us into new communities and contexts. We value and incorporate differences, framing them as sources of strength and resources rather than shame and embarrassment. We ask questions, make observations, and point out behaviors that highlight each other's contributions to the common good and how they connect to our sense of purpose or vocation.

I suspect some readers want me to provide a step-by-step "how-to" for nurturing hope. I hope what I'm communicating here is that the practices of sick children—community, power, Spirit, trust, and identity—must reflect the particularities of each time and place we seek to nurture hope. Hoping occurs in specific contexts, among specific communities, in response to specific challenges. Hope exceeds human capacities to draw on powers and realities beyond (yet glimpsed through) the material world. It participates in the slow unfolding, the ongoing manifestation, of abundance *now*. In the end, no one can tell you how to create that. We can, however, identify its markers and the practices that help make it a reality in particular lives by orienting ourselves to hope's presence and cultivating the local conditions under which it makes itself known.

IN CLOSING

Hopeful children with chronic illness find meaning in their disease, feel empowered to manage the illness, successfully integrate the chronic condition into previous identities, develop a sense of altruism related to the illness, and anticipate future achievements. They are more likely to take their medications; follow medical instructions to avoid rejecting a transplanted kidney; and manage their illness to maintain good kidney function, increase independence, avoid hospitalization, and qualify for less-demanding dialysis schedules. Without question, the health and economic benefits of nurturing hope among children with chronic illness deserve our attention.

Beyond the material benefits, there are spiritual, existential, relational, and communal reasons to become more intentional about nurturing hope among chronically ill children and adults. My conversations with sick children suggest (at least) three implications in this regard: be real, make meaning, and get specific.

First, sick children know what's going on with their bodies, their psychosocial circumstances, and their medical care; they also reflect with insight on their experiences of illness. Chronically ill children make meaning of their suffering in creative and nuanced ways. Having clear, honest, and accurate information from parents, doctors, and other members of the interdisciplinary team facilitates this process, and children with end-stage renal disease trust and value adults who know that children are responsible, knowing agents who have ever-emerging and -maturing spiritual, moral, communal, and health-related powers. Again and again, children demonstrate that they know more about their health and illness than team members tend to assume, and children say that accurate, honest medical information helps them cope. This suggests that caregivers of all types should provide specific, detailed, and developmentally appropriate information to children living with chronic illness, paying as much or more attention to their needs for information than to adults with the same disease. Relationships are not the context for the work of medicine and other types of care. Relationships are the work of medicine and other types of care. They should be distinguished by mutuality, vulnerability, respect, and humanity.

Second, grown-ups must be more intentional about cultivating transpersonal awareness among children with chronic illness, opening them to knowledge that comes to them through inner experience or authority. Such knowledge can be cultivated and accessed through intuition, imagination, creative processes, spiritual disciplines, religious insights and practices, and other forms of knowledge. This type of direct, spiritual knowing shapes children's practices of choosing trust and attending to Spirit, and it seems at work in those ordinary occasions that children describe as times they're most aware of hope. When children say illness gives them purpose, bestows special gifts or knowledge, and motivates altruistic actions, they often invoke a transpersonal wisdom that they see as authoritative. We can help children cultivate this awareness by teaching them curiosity, prayer, mindfulness, creativity, and introspection (in both the psychological and spiritual uses of the term).

Finally, my conversations with chronically ill young people clarify that hope arrives in endless, idiosyncratic ways. Reducing hope to a single phenomenon—cognition, virtue, feeling, present, past, future—can briefly be effective in some situations and for some purposes, but in the long term, humans need a multidimensional understanding of hope. Because no child or family hopes in the same ways, professionals and other caring people must work to identify the specific mix of hopeful practices already present among children and families dealing with chronic illness, and then work to amplify and strengthen those practices in relation to illness. Initially, at least, doing more of what works accomplishes more than attempting to introduce something new or different.

When I was eight years old, my family returned home late at night and discovered one of our horses giving birth under a heat lamp in the barn. Her sides heaved like bellows, and her breath came in rough blasts. Sweat darkened her coat; the straw in her stall was dark with blood and moisture. In my memory, it was a cold night, and steam swirled up from fluids that gushed from the birth canal. The foal was stuck: a single, slender leg protruded into the cold air where there should have been two. My mother took off her coat, rolled up her sleeves, and pushed the baby back into its mother. Up to her shoulder in the mare's uterus, Mom found the second front leg and repositioned the baby, pulling both legs out of the birth canal. With one last heave, the baby slipped into the world, wet and shivering. In less than an hour, the foal, licked dry by its mother, was up and nursing. The mare seemed fine. "Her body knows what to do," Mom said, "but sometimes it needs a little help."

I remember that story when I think about how hope enters the world: It knows what to do, but sometimes it needs help. When it does, we roll up our sleeves and plunge into the messiness of life to help it emerge. Is there a better metaphor than the process of birth, when hope and suffering exist simultane-ously—great pain and enormous joy at the same time?

Talking about the practices of hope (an activity Christians call *eschatology*) makes a difference in our lives together. It's relevant to how we engage each other in the constant change that characterizes life, and it demonstrates that wholeness and restoration don't wait for the end of time. Sick children remind us that we embody the reality of hope by relating to each other in ways that acknowledge, trust, and amplify the abundance flowing from the heart of life, even the parts of life that are tragic, painful, and unsettling. We aren't in control of hope. It has its own agenda and its own schedule; it's untamed and unregulated, and it doesn't always behave in the ways we prefer. Nurturing and sustaining hope aren't about achieving goals but about trusting the process by which hope manifests, having confidence in life's unfolding even when causes and conditions don't deliver what we desire. As the Quaker-Buddhist Sallie King says, "Hope is wonderful and necessary, but, if we can, we should try not to slide into cherishing expectations of how things will turn out."[6]

Many years ago, I asked a Buddhist teacher what, for Bud-dhists, correlated with Christianity's emphasis on hope. His an-swer was swift and definitive: "Courage." In Buddhism, courage requires a willingness to see life as it is, to open yourself to the world without shying or recoiling, to become vulnerable enough to act to reduce suffering in small and perhaps invisible ways. Sometimes, simply witnessing the world alleviates pain.

An ancient definition of courage is to "continue to bear with-out strength." We tend to imagine this as carrying on through exhaustion, continuing to carry something heavy despite feeling depleted and weary. But to bear something also means to give birth, to bring something into being, to push vulnerable life into the world in the midst of blood and poop and amniotic fluid. We participate in the process—our bodies know what to do—but we aren't the ones who make hope happen. It arrives on its own, inviting us to witness and midwife something new emerging, a possibility that puts boundaries on darkness and calls us into the warmth of a candlelit table promising good company and nourishing food.

PRACTICES OF HOPE AMONG CHRONICALLY ILL CHILDREN

When scholars do the type of qualitative research that informs this book, grounded theory, they eventually create an abstract "theoretical description" of each final theme that emerges from participant experiences. In this book, the themes are Realizing Connections, Claiming Power, Attending to Spirit, Choosing Trust, and Maintaining Identity as practices of hope. The appendix provides readers with the formal, theoretical description of each practice—a brief summary, if you will.

Each practice relates to four aspects of hope as described by the children: existential, sociocultural, a gift emerging from illness, and a resource carried into the illness experience. Choosing Trust and Attending to Spirit, for example, are both existential dimensions of hope, but Attending to Spirit reflects resources that children bring to the illness experience, while Choosing Trust arrives as a gift. In a similar way, Maintaining Identity, Claiming Power, and Realizing Connections are all sociocultural dimensions of hope; Maintaining Identity relates to the resources that children bring to illness, Realizing Connections is a gift that emerges from illness, and Claiming Power stands somewhere between a gift and a resource.

THEORETICAL DESCRIPTIONS OF PRACTICES

REALIZING CONNECTIONS weaves children who have end-stage renal disease into a community of mutuality and trust that assures them that they are not alone in living with the illness. This facet of hopefulness is primarily relational and agential; by making "real" their connections to others, children participate in the creation of social capital that provides resources for coping with the psychosocial, spiritual, and intra-psychic aspects of the disease. Relationships with members of the interdisciplinary treatment team are primary in this process, with boys and children older than fourteen years especially focused on connections with physicians. The illness also leads many children to develop multifaceted connections, formal and informal, to a broader community. Children particularly value connections to other children and grown-ups living with kidney disease. Connections to others are made real through conversation, visitation, consultation, and participation in daily activities; in the process, children receive (and often give) guidance, empowerment, reassurance, and encouragement. Some relationships offer children a broader vision of future possibilities despite the ongoing effects of kidney disease. This practice especially engages children of color, and it is the most prominent theme across all age groups. Because relationships generate social artifacts that can increase agency and clarify identity, realizing connections is constitutive of claiming power and maintaining identity as hopeful practices. Realizing connections represents gifts that children gain from the disease experience. It focuses on the horizontal, immanent axis of life.

CLAIMING POWER allows children with end-stage renal disease to take an active role in treatment by setting goals, advocating for themselves, choosing coping methods, and monitoring and maintaining their own health. This facet of hopefulness is primarily agential; it focuses on children's abilities to set goals, influence outcomes, access resources, and participate meaningfully as a member of the interdisciplinary team. Children claim power by refusing to be objects who passively experience the disease and its treatment; instead, they assert themselves as subjects in relation to other members of the interdisciplinary team and in relation to the effects of the disease. For some children, claiming power includes identifying and enacting strategies to control anxiety as a means of resisting the intra-psychic suffering that can accompany the illness. Choosing when and to whom to disclose illness can be one such strategy. Claiming power allows children to influence health outcomes and thereby obtain more freedom from the limitations imposed by the disease and its treatment. This practice occurs most frequently among children older than fourteen years. While boys engage this practice more prominently than girls, girls are more likely than boys to frame claiming power as a deliberate choice. Claiming power primarily represents a resource that children gain from the disease experience and focuses on the horizontal, immanent axis of life.

ATTENDING TO SPIRIT provides spiritual consolation to children with end-stage renal disease by assuring them that Spirit, as an ultimate reality, is present in their suffering and participates in the treatment process. Children of color are more likely than others to invoke this practice. Attending to Spirit manifests primarily in relational and sapiential ways, activated through religious and spiritual practices such as prayer, worship, visitation, blessing, and the reading of scripture. Some children invoke a family wisdom figure, such as a grandparent, as a spiritual guide to help them attend to Spirit. Children with end-stage renal disease tend toward an instrumental understanding of religious resources (using prayer, for example, to relieve anxiety during dialysis) but speak intimately and personally of God's availability and presence with them in the midst of illness. Prayer, especially prayer with others, is the primary way that these children connect to Spirit; this practice involves learning from, practicing with, and valuing others in formal and informal religious communities. Still, attending to Spirit focuses primarily on the vertical, transcendent horizon of life. It draws primarily on resources that children bring to the disease experience.

CHOOSING TRUST allows children with end-stage renal disease to integrate their chosen values with technical information from the interdisciplinary team and a noetic assurance about their own well-being. This facet of hopefulness is agential, relational, and resource-oriented; it can also have a transpersonal dimension, and it involves positivity, gratitude, service, awareness of death, confidence, and safety. Girls and children of color engage this practice more often than others. Choosing trust functions to enhance agency, relieve immediate intra-psychic and spiritual suffering, and generate possibilities for the future. Children seem unaware of pre-diagnosis resources and knowledge that help them cope with kidney disease; they perceive trust as evolving primarily from the team's expertise and secondarily from their own values and transpersonal awareness of a positive personal future. Among older children whose diagnosis occurred when they were young, especially White children, this integrative awareness can create a vocational desire to use their experiential wisdom to benefit other people. In this way, choosing trust moves children beyond egoic concern for their own well-being to a generative focus on the well-being of others. Finding ways to "give back" what they have received and activating a special, noetic connection with caregivers and other chronically ill patients can be significant ways that some children make meaning of their illness. This practice focuses primarily on the horizonal, immanent horizon of life; it involves both resources that children bring to the experience of disease and gifts received as part of the illness.

MAINTAINING IDENTITY reflects both the relational and psychosocial challenges that end-stage renal disease creates and the desires and efforts of children to continue to participate in activities and relationships that shaped their sense of self prior to diagnosis and treatment. This facet of hopefulness is primarily performative and agential; it focuses on what a child can do despite limitations created by the disease and treatment. Children with the disease—boys especially—are keenly aware of being different from healthy peers; behaviors and interactions that maintain pre-disease identities allow them to remain "normal" (or to become "more normal," in the words of one research partner) despite the illness. Internalized norms about being a child (established through particular sociocultural contexts) are a motivation to participate in treatment and can become a source of tension when the disease creates barriers to "being normal." Some children also discover new and positive facets of identity as they cope with the disease and seek to integrate these new self-understandings into pre-disease identities. One way that children maintain identity in the midst of treatment is by externalizing end-stage renal disease, speaking of it as an entity and force separate from and alien to themselves. This practice influences slightly more than half of the participants, disproportionately present among boys and children older than fourteen years. It focuses on the horizontal, immanent horizon of life and draws on resources that children bring to the disease experience.

A NOTE ON
METHODOLOGY

The interviews and observations at the heart of the book come from a collaborative, qualitative study I led with pediatric nephrologist Donald L. Batisky, MD.[1] We started with a small pilot study that involved twelve children in the northeastern United States; later, we embarked on a larger study with thirty-nine other children (whom we called "co-researchers" and "research partners") in the southern and southwestern United States. The second phase allowed us to test and revise the emergent theory and flesh out initial categories.

We primarily spoke with patients at hospitals where Don had privileges as a physician, but we also reached out to physicians in other locations to ensure broad geographical representation. We explored seven possibilities around the United States; in the end, three hospitals agreed to participate. One of those locations required me to become an unpaid member of its research staff (complete with an identification badge).

Each hospital's Institutional Review Board reviewed and approved the research protocol before we recruited participants. This ensured that children were protected from potential harm associated with psychosocial research. This approval was especially important because children are a vulnerable research population, and because we planned to offer a financial incentive to participate. Each hospital agreed that the incentive was reasonable and noncoercive. Participating children received a $25 gift card at the end of the interview.

Once the protocol was approved, physicians at each location introduced the project to patients (and their families) who might be thoughtful, reflective participants. Children needed to meet three criteria to participate: a diagnosis of end-stage renal disease, part of an English-speaking family, and nine to nineteen years old. If a child and family expressed interest, they met with Don, me, or both of us to talk in detail about the project, learn about potential risks, and ask questions. We selected a convenience sample at each location, that is, choosing among children readily available, and we tried to balance the number of male and female participants and ensure diverse racial-ethnic identities and treatment protocols. Parents or guardians of children younger than seventeen years provided written informed consent before the interview, while participants eighteen years and older signed the informed consent themselves. Children provided written informed assent before the interview to affirm that they had volunteered to participate. They could withdraw from the study at any point without penalty and still receive a gift card.

The interviews took place in hemodialysis units during treatment and in examination rooms during clinics for transplant recipients and peritoneal dialysis patients. Children decided whether parents would be present during the interview; most wanted to talk with us alone. I conducted most interviews, with occasional help from Don and two doctoral students.

THE CHILDREN

We interviewed fifty-one children, split evenly between sexes (49 percent, female; 51 percent, male). Most (55 percent) were fifteen years old and older; 10 percent were eleven years old or younger, with the remaining 35 percent between twelve and fourteen years old. A majority were Black and Brown (41 percent

Latino/a and 26 percent Black), with 31 percent White and 2 percent Asian. In terms of treatment, 55 percent were dialysis recipients; 43 percent had transplanted kidneys; and 2 percent returned to dialysis after a failed transplant. The largest number lived in the US Southwest (47 percent); 29 percent lived in the US South, and 24 percent in the US Northeast.

Most participants had lived with kidney disease for years, some since birth. Eighteen-year-old Amy started kidney treatment when she was six months old, and eighteen-year-old Andrew received his diagnosis two days after birth; they are the most experienced children in the study. The least experienced was sixteen-year-old Angie, who was diagnosed with kidney failure just a few weeks before our conversation.

With the exception of Angie, all of the children were used to relating to grown-up medical personnel. Children receive a lot of personal attention at the hospital; they see the same staff members on a regular basis, and they trusted us immediately. Most treated us as part of the interdisciplinary team, the ecosystem that surrounds and cares for sick children. Getting children to talk wasn't a problem; when I encountered them, they seemed comfortable, even blasé, at the hospital. Dialysis and clinics are familiar, part of daily life, like going to school or the mall. Children tended to treat the dialysis unit and examination rooms as an extension of home, welcoming us into what they saw as their space.

A few participants asked to be identified by their legal first names, but most chose a pseudonym. If a child didn't want to use their name and didn't choose a pseudonym, I selected one not already in use. While writing about participants I changed identifying details for everyone to protect their identities. All of the children quoted in the book are real, unique individuals; there are no composite characters or fictional examples.

· · · · · · · · · · · · · · · · · ·

The participants come from varied backgrounds. Some have parents who clean houses for a living; others come from politically and financially powerful families. A few live in deep poverty, going hungry so often that it's difficult to stick to diets that help their kidneys stay healthy and optimally functional. Most live in suburban or rural communities; some have parents who work multiple jobs to pay bills, while others have a stay-at-home parent who cares for them almost full time. Some are knit into large, extended families where someone always pitches in to help; others are isolated, the only child of a single parent who works long hours.

For some, life with chronic illness offers tremendous gifts. It connects them to a large, supportive community devoted to helping them achieve goals and maintain health. Others tumble through the healthcare system treated as objects, barely noticed by teachers at school, and coping alone with pain and anxiety. Some, like fifteen-year-old Calvin, try to talk to their families about the stresses of chronic illness, sharing their fears and despair, but receive responses like, "Don't whine to me; I'm not Dr. Phil," or, "You sound like a woman; man up and cope, dude" (using misogyny to shame an adolescent boy).

All of these children invited me to witness their vulnerability, fear, and suffering, as well as their joy and insight. They made it possible for me to befriend the hope that persists beneath suffering, to trust that all manner of things shall be well no matter how broken the world seems. The children in this book convinced me of the truth of the catchphrase of spiritual teacher Ram Dass: We're all just walking each other home.[2]

THE INTERVIEWS

The interviews took place in person from 2008 to 2011. The conversations lasted fifteen to sixty minutes, depending on a child's energy level and how much they wanted to say. We used Zoom H2 digital recorders to capture the conversations, assigning each child's file a unique code to protect their identities. The digital files were transcribed in Microsoft Word by paid transcriptionists whose contracts included nondisclosure agreements. We analyzed transcripts for the pilot study by hand, grouping and tacking hundreds of index cards to an upholstered wall in my office at Phillips Theological Seminary. For the second phase, I analyzed transcripts with HyperResearch 4.0.1—a more efficient if less tactile approach.

Most of the children seemed to enjoy our conversations. Dialysis can be boring—patients spend hours lying in bed or sitting in a chair—and with nothing else to do, some children talked enthusiastically and at length. They asked questions about us (Where did we go to school? Did we have kids? Had we been on dialysis? What did we do for fun?), shared jokes, and told great stories. Clinic conversations tended to be shorter; children were eager to leave, and medical staff needed the examination rooms for other patients.

Some children were more reflective and articulate than others, of course, and a few clearly agreed to an interview simply to receive a $25 gift card. (Those conversations were short, focused more on facts than meaning.) In some cases, children kept in touch after the study, using email to celebrate achievements, provide health updates, and share resources.

Interviewers usually started the conversations by asking children to share the stories of their illness. Those stories often morphed into accounts of suffering, some quite detailed. We listened to those accounts as long as children wanted to talk. When children seemed comfortable and had nothing else to share, we shifted to the actual research questions. We used a semi-structured approach to elicit children's stories and understandings of hope. The four structured questions were:

- What is hope, in your own words?
- What does it mean to have hope?

- Can you tell a story about a time you've experienced hope here at the hospital/clinic or during your illness?
- What do members of the team that takes care of you do that makes you hopeful?

We asked follow-up questions, particularly "what" and "how" questions, to elicit richer descriptions and to make sure we grasped what children were communicating. We tried to understand behavior and situations as the children understood them, learn about their lives from their perspectives, and adopt their definitions and interpretations of the things they talked about. Over time, attempting to be more concrete (especially with younger children), I added a question like, "Suppose you met a kid who's just been diagnosed and starting dialysis. What would you tell them about hope and how to be hopeful with kidney disease?" I asked follow-up questions to clarify what the child thought was important or useful about their advice, and why.

FROM INTERVIEWS TO DATA

In creating and conducting the study, we used constructionist grounded theory as a methodological approach. In this approach, data collection, data analysis, and theory building happen simultaneously; they overlap and mutually influence each other. The words of children drove data collection, analysis, and interpretation from the earliest days of the study to help create a theory of pediatric hope in chronic illness that reflected their experiences as closely as possible. We used purposeful sampling to ensure diverse racial, ethnic, developmental, and treatment perspectives, and we used strategic sampling to generate and saturate emerging categories, codes, and theories.

The goal of grounded theory research is to propose a theory "grounded in" (and accountable to) the words of participants. The theory emerges as researchers identify common themes in the data that illuminate the issues people are attempting to understand, cope with, and resolve. As researchers label interview data with labels, then group related labels into broader themes, the emerging themes and categories become increasingly abstract. By the time a researcher proposes a theory, what it articulates is necessarily more conceptual and general than the concrete details of people's experiences expressed in interviews. But the resulting theory should connect all of the individual stories, telling a life-like story that sufficiently accounts for behaviors, experiences, and interpretations that participants share across contexts. When participants read the results of a grounded theory study, they should recognize their experience even if they wouldn't use those specific words. The researcher wants participants to say: "Yes! That's what it's like!"

This approach assumes that knowledge doesn't exist, waiting to be discovered, but is constructed through relationship. Grounded theory is particularly suited to exploring meaning and subjective experience; its value is its descriptive and generative power rather than its ability to predict what will happen or generalize to other settings or populations. It prioritizes patterns, connections, and understanding, not explanation. It's an imaginative interpretation with pragmatic uses; it allows us to imagine possibilities, establish connections, and identify new questions.[3] It seeks to be credible, original, and useful. It should resonate with people whose circumstances are similar to those of participants, and it should help make a better world for them.

As these processes occurred, we constantly compared what we were hearing and seeing from different children; we also compared the content from my observational memos about the clinics and dialysis units where interviews took place. These memos recorded not only observations but also my thoughts, ideas, and questions as I sought to make sense of what the children said. Sometimes Don and I recorded conversations over coffee or between interviews to capture our evolving thoughts about the project; those recordings were transcribed into research memos and became part of the data.

FROM DATA TO BOOK

Once data has been collected, analyzed, and interpreted, it should be shared with people who can benefit from what is learned. Don and I presented our work—primarily based on the pilot study—to scholars, researchers, chaplains, and medical personnel through journal articles, book chapters, workshops, and lectures from Florida to Ohio to California. We also established the Children's Hope Initiative to make this early work available to parents, children, religious leaders, and others. Changes in my personal and professional life after active fieldwork—interviewing children and hanging around dialysis units and transplant clinics—led to a long period away from the data, reflecting on what I had learned about hope.

Over time, mostly during summers when I wasn't teaching, I began to analyze and reanalyze all of the data. I read and reread transcripts, compared the experiences of children from different settings, coded and recoded interviews, and reviewed memos I had written about each site. As I combed through twenty years of files, resources, and the drafts of earlier projects about hope that did not include empirical research, I gained a richer understanding of what the children were saying and how it connected (or not) to other research on the topic.

Software helped me identify previously unnoticed connections and nuances in the data. In particular, I saw different emphases between sexes, across ages, and among racial-ethnic identities. Arranging data visually with mind-maps further clarified relationships among the children's ideas and experiences, which led me to write new descriptions of each practice to clarify and nuance their contours. Gradually, I realized I needed to write a book about the children and what they taught me about hope—both because the information was important and because I owed these research partners so much.

While writing, I honored the norms of critical ethnography and autoethnography to weave together the children's stories with research from multiple academic disciplines so that their experiences shed light on broader cultural phenomena. What happens day by day to children with chronic illness can illuminate cultural meanings of sickness, health, ability, disability, chronic illness, and more in ways that are useful to others.

ACKNOWLEDGMENTS

This book is dedicated to (and possible because of a long friendship and collaboration with) Donald L. Batisky, MD, professor of pediatrics and associate dean for admissions and special
programs at the University of Cincinnati College of Medicine.
Don and I started researching pediatric hope together in 2008.
At the time, he served as professor and director of admissions at
the School of Medicine at the Ohio State University. During most
of our collaboration, he was professor of pediatric nephrology
and director of the Pediatric Hypertension Program at the School
of Medicine of Emory University, as well as executive director of
the PreHealth Mentoring Office at the university's College of Arts
and Sciences. We have been close friends for more than fifteen
years, presenting together at conferences, co-authoring journal
articles, and receiving a collaborative grant to expand our research. More recently, Don generously read the book manuscript,
correcting my misunderstandings of the medical dimensions of
end-stage renal disease and offering useful suggestions. I am
profoundly grateful for his support, critique, and friendship.

Three US medical centers supported and facilitated our research. I am grateful to the physicians, nurses, administrators,
and other staff members who welcomed us and helped me understand the intricacies of life with kidney disease. To protect the
identities of the children with whom I talked, I am not naming

the specific medical centers or staff members that hosted our work. Yet I am deeply indebted to each individually and to all of them together. They provide evidence that angels walk among us.

Many scholars, practitioners, students, and religious communities shaped my thinking about childhood hope. In particular, I am grateful to the Society for Pastoral Theology, which invited me to present my work-in-progress in 2010; the society's Working Group on Religious Practices and Pastoral Research, which engaged my work in 2009; the *Journal of Pastoral Theology* and the online journal *Childhood and Religion*, which published early manuscripts from the pilot study; the Children and Religion Unit of the American Academy of Religion; the Midwest Pediatric Kidney Association; the Third Triennial Children's Spirituality Conference: Christian Perspectives; Kevin Lawson, editor of *Understanding Children's Spirituality: Theology, Research, and Practice*; the Spiritual Care Collaborative; the Taos Institute Associate's Council; the Center for Health Professions Education, Hebert School of Medicine, Uniformed Services University of the Health Sciences in Bethesda, Maryland; Claremont School of Theology, Claremont, California; Phillips Theological Seminary in Tulsa; All Church Home for Children in Fort Worth; Harvard Avenue Christian Church in Tulsa; Claremont Presbyterian Church in Claremont, California; Hillcrest Medical Center in Tulsa; Nationwide Children's Hospital in Columbus, Ohio; St. Mark's Meditation Center in Washington, DC; and Texas Medical Center in Houston. Lerrill White, former director of clinical pastoral education at St. Luke's Episcopal Hospital in Houston, invited me to offer a week of teaching on hope nearly fifteen years ago. Karen-Marie Yust of Union Presbyterian Seminary and the late Don Browning of the University of Chicago wrote letters of support for a grant application to expand the pilot project.

Research funding came from the Lilly Theological Grants Program of the Association of Theological Schools and from the Medical College of the Ohio State University. The Taos Institute supported the establishment of the Children's Hope Initiative, and Amanda Enayati served as a researcher and writer for that project. The trustees, president, dean, and faculty of Claremont School of Theology provided a research leave in spring 2021 that allowed me to make progress on the first draft of the manuscript. Steven J. Durning, director of the Center for Health Professions Education and vice chair of the department of medicine, supported the completion of the book after I joined the faculty of the Uniformed Services University of the Health Sciences in 2022.

My curiosity about pediatric hope sparked during a short tenure as chaplain at Cook Children's Medical Center in Fort Worth. Later, as a doctoral student, I studied pediatric care in the classroom (and beyond) with the Rev. Ann Miller, PhD, the hospital's director of pastoral care. Now retired, Ann was a founding member of the Pediatric Chaplains Network. My final paper for her course at Brite Divinity School planted the seed for this project. Andy Lester's work on the pastoral dimensions of hope informed my early understandings, and Carolyn Osiek and Elaine Robinson, former colleagues at Brite Divinity School, engaged in helpful conversation when the project was just an idea. The late C. R. Snyder at the University of Kansas engaged me in virtual conversation about his cognitive model of hope. Sallie Sampsell Watson and John McMillan provided feedback on drafts of a precursor project. Amy Miller Caldwell, editorial director at Beacon Press, shaped the book significantly, and Susan Lumenello, managing editor at Beacon, provided consummate copyediting (making me appear smarter than I am). Don Batisky, Ben Bidwell, Burke Gerstenschlager, and David Lott commented on the proposal.

My colleagues Kathy Black, David Lott, and Josh Morris read drafts of the manuscript; Josh also provided research assistance during his PhD work at Claremont School of Theology. Early research assistance came from Jamie Phelps and Molly Taylor at Brite Divinity School and Brenda Fletchall at Phillips Theological

Seminary. Minhwan Song and Krista Wuertz served as research assistants during their PhD work at Claremont School of Theology, and Min did heavy lifting on citations, formatting, and other tasks during the final stages of the manuscript. Michael Cook and Isaac Arthur assisted with research interviews during their doctoral studies at Emory University. Medical student Nicole Holly helped me describe the vascular system accurately when she unwisely sat next to me on a Southwest flight from Phoenix to Portland. The community at St. Andrew's Abbey in Valyermo, California, especially Father Francis Benedict, OSB, provided space and sustenance for writing. Sheryn Scott loaned her cabin for writing and reflection, and David Gutterman and I wrote together virtually each week from January to August 2021. Photographer Brian Hernandez asked regularly about the book's progress and provided a sounding board for the ups and downs of writing. Since 2007, my virtual writing group has provided weekly accountability and encouragement; these days its members are Emily Askew (Lexington Theological Seminary), Eileen Campbell-Reed (Union Theological Seminary in the City of New York), Mary Moschella (Yale Divinity School), Rochelle Robins (Academy of Jewish Religion-California), Tim Robinson (Brite Divinity School), and Janet Schaller (private practice, Memphis).

Ultimately, I am most grateful to and for Karee Galloway, my wife and partner, and our son, Ben. They collaborate in the hope at the center of my life, providing humor, support, sustenance, appropriate ego deflation, and remarkable tolerance with unmerited generosity and unearned patience.

NOTES

AUTHOR'S NOTE

1. Duane R. Bidwell, *When One Religion Isn't Enough: The Lives of Spiritually Fluid People* (Boston: Beacon Press, 2018), 2–3.

2. See Arthur P. Bochner and Carolyn Ellis, *Evocative Ethnography: Writing Lives and Telling Stories* (New York: Routledge, 2016).

CHAPTER 1: TETHERED

1. Peggy Way, *Created by God: Pastoral Care for All God's People* (St. Louis: Chalice Press), 37.

CHAPTER 2: REALIZING CONNECTIONS

1. Pamela D. Couture, *Seeing Children, Seeing God: A Practical Theology of Children and Poverty* (Nashville: Abingdon Press, 2000), 29–35.

2. Couture, *Seeing Children, Seeing God*, 37.

3. Okba F. Ahmed, Omar M. Hamodat, Fahmi H. Kakamad, Rabea S. Abduljabbar, Abdulwahid M. Salih, Diyar A. Omar, Mohammed Q. Mustafa, Marwan N. Hassan, Shvan H. Mohammed, Tomas M. Mikael, Kayhan A. Najar, and Dahat A. Hussen, "Outcomes of Arteriovenous Fistula for Hemodialysis in Pediatric Age Group," *Annals of Medicine and Surgery* 72 (2021): 1–3, https://doi.org/10.1016/j.amsu.2021.103100; Deepa H. Chand, Rudolph P. Valentini, and Elaine S. Kamil, "Hemodialysis Vascular Access Options in Pediatrics: Considerations for Patients and Practitioners," *Pediatric Nephrology* 24 (2009): 1121–28.

4. Jerome Groopman, *The Anatomy of Hope: How People Prevail in the Face of Illness* (New York: Random House, 2004), 185.

5. Alan E. Lewis, "Hope," *A Dictionary of Pastoral Care*, ed. Alastair V. Campbell (New York: Crossroad, 1987), 116.

6. Christopher Lasch, *The True and Only Heaven: Progress and Its Critics* (New York: Norton, 1991), 530.

7. Hal S. Shorey, C. R. Snyder, Xiangdong Yang, and Michael R. Lewin, "The Role of Hope as a Mediator in Recollected Parenting, Adult Attachment, and Mental Health," *Journal of Social and Clinical Psychology* 22, no. 6 (2003): 686, 705.

CHAPTER 3: CLAIMING POWER

1. Glenn H. Bock, Edward J. Ruley, and Michael P. Moore, *A Parent's Guide to Kidney Disorders*, University of Minnesota Guides to Birth and Childhood Disorders (Minneapolis: University of Minnesota Press, 1993), 66.

2. See Bonnie J. Miller-McLemore, *Let the Children Come: Reimagining Childhood from a Christian Perspective* (San Francisco: Jossey-Bass, 2004), 13–18.

3. Miller-McLemore, *Let the Children Come*, 137–60.

4. Sandra Amaral and Rachel Patzer, "Disparities, Race/Ethnicity and Access to Pediatric Kidney Transplantation," *Current Opinion in Nephrology and Hypertension* 22, no. 3 (2013): 336–43, https://doi.org/10.1097/MNH.0b013e32835fe55b.

5. Amaral and Patzer, "Disparities, Race/Ethnicity and Access to Pediatric Kidney Transplantation."

6. Elaine Ku, Charles E. McCulloch, Barbara A. Grimes, and Kirsten L. Johansen, "Racial and Ethnic Disparities in Survival of Children with ESRD," *Journal of the American Society of Nephrology: JASN* 28, no. 5 (2017), 1584–91, https://doi.org/10.1681/ASN.2016060706.

7. Amaral and Patzer, "Disparities, Race/Ethnicity and Access to Pediatric Kidney Transplantation."

8. Amaral and Patzer, "Disparities, Race/Ethnicity and Access to Pediatric Kidney Transplantation."

9. International Health Conference, "Constitution of the World Health Organization. 1946," *Bulletin of the World Health Organization* 80, no. 12 (2002): 983–84, https://apps.who.int/iris/handle/10665/268688.

10. Cynthia Bourgeault, *Mystical Hope: Trusting in the Mercy of God* (Cambridge, MA: Cowley Publications, 2001), 9.

11. Dr. Sami Schalk (@DrSamiSchalk), Twitter, January 12, 2022, https://twitter.com/DrSamiSchalk/status/1481259420751441921?s=20.

CHAPTER 4: ATTENDING TO SPIRIT

1. See Kenneth I. Pargament, *The Psychology of Religion and Coping: Theory, Research, Practice* (New York: Guilford, 1997).

2. Eugene C. Roehlkepartain, Peter L. Benson, Peter C. Scales, Lisa Kimball, and Pamela E. King, *With Their Own Voices: A Global Exploration of How Today's Young People Experience and Think About Spiritual Development* (Minneapolis: Search Institute Center for Spiritual Development in Childhood and Adolescence, 2008).

3. Roehlkepartain, Benson, Scales, Kimball, and King, *With Their Own Voices*.

4. Laura H. Lipman and Hugh McIntosh, "The Demographics of Spirituality and Religiosity Among Youth: International and U.S. Patterns," *ChildTrends Research Brief* (Washington, DC, 2010); Pew Research Center, "Religious Landscape Study," 2015, https://www.pewresearch.org/religion/religious-landscape-study/racial-and-ethnic-composition; Pew Research Center, *U.S. Public Becoming Less Religious*, November 3, 2015, https://www.pewresearch.org/religion/2015/11/03/u-s-public-becoming-less-religious; Eugene Roehlkepartain, Peter L. Benson, Pamela E. King, and Linda Wagener, "Spiritual Development in Childhood and Adolescence: Moving to the Scientific Mainstream," in *The Handbook of Spiritual Development in Childhood and Adolescence*, ed. Eugene Roehlkepartain, Pamela E. King, and Linda Wagener (Thousand Oaks, CA: Sage, 2006), 1–15.

5. Andrea L. Canada, George Fitchett, Patricia E. Murphy, Kevin Stein, Kenneth Portier, Corinne Crammer, and Amy H. Peterman, "Racial/Ethnic Differences in Spiritual Well-Being Among Cancer Survivors," *Journal of Behavioral Medicine* 36 (2013): 441–53, https://doi.org/10.1007/s10865-012-9439-8.

6. Joan Chittister, *Wisdom Distilled from the Daily: Living the Rule of St. Benedict Today* (San Francisco: HarperCollins, 1990), 4.

7. Chittister, *Wisdom Distilled from the Daily*, 5.

8. Chittister, *Wisdom Distilled from the Daily*, 5.

9. Daniel S. Schipani, "Pastoral and Spiritual Care in Multifaith Contexts," in *Teaching for a Multifaith World*, ed. Eleazar S. Fernandez (Eugene, OR: Pickwick, 2017), 124–46.

10. Simon Lasair, "A Narrative Approach to Spirituality and Spiritual Care in Health Care," *Journal of Religion and Health* 59 (2020): 1524–40.

11. Steven J. Sandage, David Rupert, George S. Stavros, and Nancy G. Devor, *Relational Spirituality in Psychotherapy: Healing Suffering and Promoting Growth* (Washington, DC: American Psychological Association, 2020).

12. Akbar Darvishi, Masoumeh Otaghi, and Shahram Mami, "The Effectiveness of Spiritual Therapy on Spiritual Well-Being, Self-Esteem

and Self-Efficacy in Patients on Hemodialysis," *Journal of Religion and Health* 59 (2020): 277–88, https://doi.org/10.1007/s10943-018-00750-1.

13. Kenneth Pargament, Margaret Feuille, and Donna Burdzy, "The Brief RCOPE: Current Psychometric Status of a Short Measure of Religious Coping," *Religions* 2, no. 1 (2011): 51–76, https://doi.org/10.3390/rel2010051.

14. Pargament, Feuille, and Burdzy, "The Brief RCOPE."

15. Pargament, Feuille, and Burdzy, "The Brief RCOPE."

16. Pargament, Feuille, and Burdzy, "The Brief RCOPE."

17. Pargament, Feuille, and Burdzy, "The Brief RCOPE."

18. Darvishi, Otaghi, and Mami, "The Effectiveness of Spiritual Therapy."

19. Darvishi, Otaghi, and Mami, "The Effectiveness of Spiritual Therapy."

20. James Garbarino, Nancy Dubrow, Kathleen Kostelny, and Carole Pardo, *Children in Danger: Coping with the Consequences of Community Violence*, Jossey-Bass Social and Behavioral Science Series (San Francisco: Jossey-Bass, 1998).

CHAPTER 5: CHOOSING TRUST

1. John Templeton Foundation Board of Trustees, "Generosity: Is It Really Better to Give Than to Receive?" Character Virtue Development, John Templeton Foundation, https://www.templeton.org/news/generosity-is-it-really-better-to-give-than-receive, accessed November 1, 2022.

2. Willie James Jennings, *After Whiteness: An Education in Belonging* (Grand Rapids, MI: Eerdmans, 2020).

3. Cortland Dahl, "How to Create a Sense of Purpose, According to Science: Training Your Mind to Find Meaning in Everyday Life," "Elemental" section, *Medium*, March 31, 2021, https://elemental.medium.com/how-to-create-a-sense-of-purpose-according-to-science-17ba921e1e6e; Cortland J. Dahl, Christine D. Wilson-Mendenhall, and Richard J. Davidson, "The Plasticity of Well-Being: A Training-Based Framework for the Cultivation of Human Flourishing," *Proceedings of the National Academy of the Sciences of the United States* 117, no. 51 (December 2020), https://doi.org/doi/10.1073/pnas.2014859117.

4. Kenneth J. Doka, *Counseling Individuals with Life-Threatening Illness* (New York: Springer, 2009).

5. Robert G. Sacco, "Re-Envisaging the Eight Developmental Stages of Erik Erikson: Fibonacci Life-Chart Method (FLCM),"

Journal of Educational and Developmental Psychology 3, no. 1 (2013): 140–46, https://doi.org/10.5539/jedp.v3n1p140.

6. Dahl, Wilson-Mendenhall, and Davidson, "The Plasticity of Well-Being."

7. Dahl, Wilson-Mendenhall, and Davidson, "The Plasticity of Well-Being."

8. Joanna Macy and Chris Johnstone, *Active Hope: How to Face the Mess We're in Without Going Crazy* (Novato, CA: New World Library, 2012), 233.

9. Christina A. Kilby, "The Gift of Fearlessness: A Buddhist Framework for the Protection of Vulnerable Populations Under International Humanitarian Law," *Contemporary Buddhism* (June 2, 2022): 1–13, https://doi.org/10.1080/14639947.2022.2038027.

CHAPTER 6: MAINTAINING IDENTITY

1. Michael White, *Maps of Narrative Practice* (New York: Norton, 2007).

2. Mary Catherine Bateson, *Composing a Further Life: The Age of Active Wisdom* (New York: Vintage, 2010), 95.

3. World Health Organization, *Promoting Mental Health: Concepts, Emerging Evidence, Practice (Summary Report)* (Geneva: World Health Organization, 2004).

CHAPTER 7: LEARNING FROM CHILDREN

1. Kathleen J. Greider, *Much Madness Is Divinest Sense: Wisdom in Memoirs of Soul-Suffering* (Cleveland: Pilgrim, 2007).

2. David H. Jensen, *Graced Vulnerability: A Theology of Childhood* (Cleveland: Pilgrim Press, 2005).

3. Kathy Charmaz, *Good Days, Bad Days: The Self and Chronic Illness in Time* (New Brunswick, NJ: Rutgers University Press, 1993), 6.

4. Marlene Mayra Ferreras, *Insurrectionist Wisdoms: Toward a North American Indigenized Pastoral Theology*, Environment and Religion in Feminist-Womanist, Queer, and Indigenous Perspectives (Lanham, MD: Lexington Books, 2022), 168, 211.

5. Pamela Couture, *Child Poverty: Love, Justice, and Social Responsibility* (St. Louis: Chalice Press, 2007).

6. Sallie B. King, "Hope in Engaged Buddhism," in *Hope: A Form of Delusion? Buddhist and Christian Perspectives*, ed. Elizabeth Harris (Sankt Ottilien, Germany: EOS Editions Sankt Ottilien, 2013), 169.

A NOTE ON METHODOLOGY

1. Duane R. Bidwell and Donald L. Batisky, "Abundance in Finitude: An Exploratory Study of Children's Accounts of Hope in Chronic Illness," *Journal of Pastoral Theology* 19, no. 1 (2009): 38–59; Duane R. Bidwell, "Eschatology and Childhood Hope: Reflections from Work in Progress," *Journal of Pastoral Theology* 20, no. 2 (2010): 109–27; Duane R. Bidwell and Donald L. Batisky, "Identity and Wisdom as Elements of a Spirituality of Hope Among Children with End-Stage Renal Disease," *Journal of Childhood and Religion* 2 (2011); Duane R. Bidwell and Donald L. Batisky, "The Roles of Identity and Wisdom in a Spirituality of Hope Among Children with End-Stage Renal Disease," in *Understanding Children's Spirituality: Theology, Research, and Practice*, ed. Kevin E. Lawson (Eugene, OR: Cascade, 2012), 399–418.

2. Ram Dass, *Walking Each Other Home: Conversations on Loving and Dying* (Boulder, CO: Sounds True, 2018).

3. Kathy Charmaz, *Constructing Grounded Theory: A Practical Guide Through Qualitative Analysis* (Los Angeles: Sage, 2006), 135.